Praise

"I was really struggling to keep my mask on at night, and sleep apnea was very debilitating for me. I was always tired, depressed, had short term memory loss, and overall quality of life was poor. I discovered Dr. Petkus, and started doing the breathing exercises. This one change completely turned my sleep apnea around! I went from over 30 episodes an hour to less than 1 episode per hour. Last weekend, I even played soccer for two hours! This has been an answer to a prayer!"

— **Mitch, 67 from Ontario, Canada**

"I am celebrating mentally and physically 'rising from the ashes.' I feel completely empowered to effect the change that will help heal and sustain me. I am celebrating an improvement in my sleep. I am also beginning to see an improvement in my cognition. I am beginning to multi-task again and do things that I was not capable of doing within the last few years."

— **Sarah, 52, from Charlotte, North Carolina**

"I started doing Dr P's exercises, and adjusting my diet. They actually worked and very quickly. I'm still using the cpap but I think I will stop in a week's time. Absolutely life changing. Thank you. Dr. Petkus."

— **Mark, 57, from Houston, Texas**

"I am now aware of things about my breathing that I never knew and I am a doctor! My pulmonologist has been very condescending and just told me that I needed the CPAP. This has been a real eye-opener for me and I'm noticing immediate benefits with easier sleep and less snoring!"

— **Melissa, 52, from Salt Lake City, Utah**

"Before your program, I tried going without a CPAP, but it never worked for me. Now, after working with you, I can't overstate the joy of sleeping without a CPAP."

— **Trevor, 49, from Fayetteville, Arkansas**

Sleep Apnea Solution

Sleep Apnea Solution

Less Snoring, Less CPAP,
Just Sleep

Dylan Petkus, MD, MPH, MS

DINOSB
-PRESS-

DinoSB Press
Tallahassee, Florida

Paperback ISBN: 978-1-7360587-6-3
eBook ISBN: 978-1-7360587-7-0
Library of Congress Control Number: 2024917815

About the Author

Dylan Petkus, MD, MPH, MS attended Pennsylvania State University for a Bachelor of Science in Kinesiology. Upon graduation, he received a research Fellowship award for a PhD program at the same university. However, wanting to be more involved in helping people directly, he decided to leave early with his Master's degree in Physiology and authored several papers. Then, he attended the University of Miami Miller School of Medicine in Florida and earned two degrees: a Master's in Public Health and a Medical Degree. Due to the traffic on I-95, he desired to work in a rural area and went to Tallahassee, Florida for residency in Family Medicine. Now, he works with people remotely all over the world to overcome sleep apnea with natural lifestyle solutions. His primary hobbies include writing "About the Author" sections in the third person, lame jokes (such as this), and having fun outdoors with his wife, three dogs, and three cats.

For my beloved wife, my constant source of love, strength and support. Thank you for being by my side every step of this journey.

To my amazing patients over the years who inspired me to find a better solution. This book is for you.

Hi Mom. Hi Dad.

Table of Contents

Who is this for?

This book is for anyone with confirmed or suspected obstructive sleep apnea. Or you may be dealing with snoring. Either way, this book is for you.

If you're using continuous positive airway pressure (CPAP) or a similar device right now, then this book is also for you. What you'll learn here will help you get better sleep if you're using one. And, with the guidance of your healthcare provider, you can start to reduce your reliance on a CPAP as appropriate.

Get The Sleep Apnea Solution Jumpstart

Dealing with sleep apnea alone can be daunting. That's why I created The Sleep Apnea Solution Jumpstart, a bonus email course designed to make tackling sleep apnea easier.

This course is designed for people like you who are ready to take action and gain control over their sleep apnea. By signing up below, you'll gain access to:

- **Exclusive Articles and Videos**: Simplified lessons to help you understand and apply key concepts.
- **Q&A Sessions with Dr. Dylan Petkus**: Ask questions and get personalized guidance on your sleep apnea journey.
- **Exclusive Assessments**: Gain insights into your unique sleep apnea challenges.
- **Audio Tracks of Breathing Exercises**: Practice and master these techniques anytime, anywhere.

- **Comprehensive Action Checklists**: Step-by-step guides to ensure you don't miss anything on your path to better sleep.

The Sleep Apnea Solution Jumpstart is your fast track to taking control of your sleep apnea. Use the link below to gain your exclusive, complimentary course and jumpstart your journey to better sleep today!

TheSleepApneaSolution.com/jumpstart

Join The Movement & Connect with Me!

I know that technically we just met, and even then, it's through the pages of this book rather than in person. Nonetheless, I'd like to extend a special invitation for you to join our private online community on Facebook.

Why Join Our Movement?

As we both know, how we approach sleep apnea is failing millions of people. Yet, everywhere you turn, someone tries to strap you onto a CPAP that you don't want. That's why we need to band together to overcome sleep apnea once and for all.

Also, throughout this book, I'll provide links to discussions and action steps designed to help you implement the beneficial strategies even more effectively.

Our group is focused on being a valuable resource for your journey. Here's everything included in the group as a complimentary bonus for being an owner of this book:

- **Exclusive Access:** Gain entry to valuable discussion threads and resources linked throughout the book.
- **Supportive Community:** Connect with like-minded individuals who are on the same journey, sharing experiences and tips.
- **Direct Interaction:** Participate in discussions that deepen your understanding of the book's content.

More importantly, I don't want you to get excited about a specific discussion thread, click it, and then realize you can't access it until you're a member of the group (unfortunately, I don't make the rules of Facebook; you can take that up with Mark Zuckerberg).

So, save yourself the frustration and join us by using this link (put it in your browser or touch/click if you have the e-book):

TheSleepApneaSolution.com/community

For an easier way, even if you're not tech savvy, you may use the camera on your phone to scan this QR code. **All you need to do is use your phone's camera to focus on the code below, and you'll see a link pop up on your phone.**

Introduction:

Hi! It's Dylan Petkus, MD, MPH, MS here.

I don't usually include all my academic degrees when introducing myself via text, but it's related to the first point I want to make in this book.

Despite having spent seven years at graduate level education (and that's not even including residency), I am highly against "intellectual hoarding." In fact, when I was in graduate school, I was aiming for a PhD (I left with a master's instead). The big reason for leaving early was that I felt none of my efforts would ever allow me to directly impact the lives of people dealing with real problems in the real world.

Don't get me wrong. Academic research is essential. You will find that I cite research throughout this book (as I should). That's because not only are big studies involving hundreds of people important but so are the shrimps running on treadmills somewhere (unfortunately, shrimps on treadmills are not relevant for sleep apnea as of 2024).

Instead of gathering facts, I am focused on ***information*** that leads to ***informed action*** (I don't think I'm clever enough to be the first person to discover this wordplay). I'm sure you're also guilty of piling up books on your bookshelf, e-reader, or computer that haven't been read (and if you're reading this, then you've broken that habit—so, great job!). You may have even read a book and thought the action steps were cool. But you didn't apply them thoroughly.

That's why this book is designed to be highly actionable.

I've been in your sleepy, brain-fogged shoes. I know what it's like to have a thought come to mind only to vanish a minute later. I've had my extensive to-do list stifle my unmotivated, tired brain to the point of paralysis and inaction.

I am not going to bore you with 200 pages of backstory (but maybe 30 pages). I'm not writing pages upon pages of information that has a poor squeeze-to-juice ratio (that's the fanciest way to say "the juice ain't worth the squeeze" or that the information won't change your results much).

However, if we only seek to understand and not apply anything, then we're in trouble. The reality is that this book *itself* will do nothing for your sleep apnea. *The magic is you applying what you have learned!*

You will get the best results by following the steps laid out in the book. Some of them will make sense to you. Some of them won't really click with you right away. Either way, do them all! *If you pick and choose your action steps, you don't get to pick your results!*

Lastly, do not make this an "I'll start on Monday" health adventure. There will never be a time in your life to focus on your health. In fact, it is better to focus on your health while you have life going on. That's because real, lasting change happens when you integrate healthy habits into your everyday life, not when you isolate them to a specific time or circumstance.

By focusing on your health amid the challenges of work, piano recitals, and even vacation, you develop the skills, resilience, and adaptability needed to maintain your well-being for the long haul.

That's why the perfect time to start is *right now*, while embracing the imperfections of life. Now, don't worry. We're not going to make drastic changes on the first day. This is all designed for a tired person with a full-time job, four kids, two dogs, and three cats.

So, put aside "doomsday news" for a bit (the earth will still be falling apart when you tune back in), catch yourself while scrolling on social media, and focus on you. You deserve it. The people around you deserve it. The moments when you can achieve, be fully present, and experience genuine joy and fulfillment are all waiting for you.

Here's your first mini-action step:

Decide when you'll carve out twenty minutes to go over one chapter daily. (I'm being generous with the time commitment if you need to review anything.)

Seriously... when?

Is it in the morning?

During lunchtime?

At 7 p.m. every night?

Write it on a sticky note. Tell your partner (Seriously, tell them what you're up to—that will help tremendously).

The best time is whenever you'll be the most consistent!

(Remember what you've consistently done when you have time to squeeze it in? Me neither!)

So, decide when you will set aside the time for yourself!

Get The Sleep Apnea Solution Jumpstart

In the theme of action, if you have not gotten access to the Sleep Apnea Solution Jumpstart, then I'd highly recommend you do so now with the link below. You will get a lots of incredibly valuable resources such as:
- Exclusive articles & videos
- Q&A sessions with me
- Assessments
- Downloadable audio tracks for the breathing exercises
- And easy-action checklists for the healthy lifestyle changes. Just use this link below:

TheSleepApneaSolution.com/jumpstart

Chapter 1
Why We're Here

We're all here for the same reason: ***something happened.***

I'm not only talking about sleep apnea because that nuisance (which is an understatement) has been going on for a while if you're reading this. Even if you've been recently diagnosed, the chances are it has been brewing for months or even years.

If you're human like me, we had a similar path. I was going about my life not thinking much about my health. Now, don't get me wrong, I would work out and eat relatively healthy foods, but I spent more of my time focused on things that excited me.

I was pursuing professional goals in academic research at The Pennsylvania State University. I was spending quality time being active out on the hiking trails nearby. And I was having fun with family and friends.

But then things started to change. At first, I started to have a bad night of sleep here and there. Luckily, coffee (the sweet nectar of the just-keep-pushing gods), allowed me to keep plowing through work and all my other obligations.

But, over time, the worsening sleep crept up on me. What started out as bad sleep one or two times a week became most nights. Then, every night became a struggle. I'd be waking up three, four, even five times a night. I dreaded sleep so much I started to have recurring dreams that I was a sardine trying to break out of a can. (Luckily the smell didn't follow me out of the dream.)

As unpleasant as that was, I didn't really think much of it at the time. It was just my normal. I pushed through everything from work to Thanksgiving dinner with my family. Figure 1 illustrates how much I wanted to use the Thanksgiving mashed potatoes as a pillow.

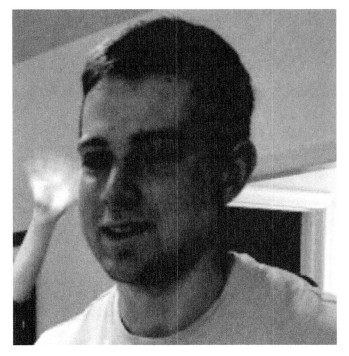

Figure 1-1: Dylan longs for a fluffy, white pillow

When I realized something was definitely amiss with my sleep, that's what pushed me to finally see my doctor. After talking with him, I ended up getting set up with a sleep study. So, I found myself there with wires sprouting from my head like some human circuit board.

When my results came back and I had my follow up appointment, I heard the fateful words, *"You have obstructive sleep apnea."* My heart sank as if I'd been given a life sentence.

Ultimately, I ended up trying out the route of the CPAP. I had my initial titration study in the sleep lab (which was a blast, as Figure 2 captures).

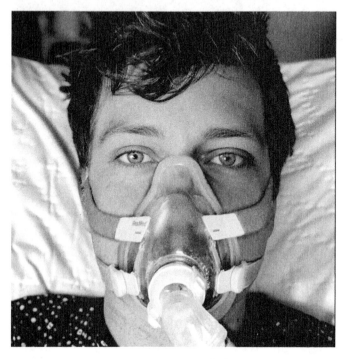

Figure 1-2: Enjoying an exhilarating CPAP titration study

After that exhausting night, I had my own to try. I hesitated that night, filled with dread. But I had no choice. I just wanted to not feel so tired all the time.

I awoke the next day feeling like I'd slept even worse. This was massively frustrating as I wrestled throughout the night with the discomfort of the mask and the noise of the machine. That's what brought me to the decision to refuse this contraption as my only answer. Even if I found a way to be more comfortable with it at night, the thought of being dependent on the CPAP for the rest of my life was debilitating.

So, I decided to go down every rabbit hole I could find. I went to my local dentist and ENT doctor, who suggested expensive devices and procedures that would "*hopefully help a bit.*"

Instead of taking that gamble, I took to the internet in search of a better solution. I scoured Amazon looking for anything that seemed promising. I crammed plastic mouth guards in that only made sleep more uncomfortable. I tried exercise gadgets only to have a sore mouth and very little sleep improvement. I resolved not to keep relying on the next thing Amazon suggested for me to buy or on conventional medicine's opinion on devices and medications.

Life continued to be a struggle as I plodded through my journey to overcome my sleep apnea. I was still waking up several times a night and spending my days exhausted. Work was impossible at that point. I was in a PhD program which demanded high-level intellectual output.

Outside of work, my personal life suffered too. I used to enjoy hiking and playing sports, but the constant fatigue left me with no energy for these activities. Social gatherings became a rare occurrence, as I often found myself too tired to engage with friends and family. Weekends, which once were filled with adventures and fun, turned into recovery days where I just tried to catch up on rest.

I got used to pushing through the days like this. I was more caught up in trying to cope with life than to fully devote myself to fixing this problem as if my life depended on it.

But then one day, I had a wake-up call (and I'm not talking about my alarm clock). I was supposed to do some experiments on rare samples for a big research project that my coworker had spent years collecting. But because I was always so tired and out of it, I mixed up the tubes and did the wrong tests. In just a few hours, I had ruined years of hard work.

My boss was furious and said I was lazy and didn't care about the team. My coworker, who had tears in their eyes from being so upset, couldn't even look at me. I felt awful and ashamed. I was scared of getting fired and felt terrible for letting everyone down after they had trusted me with such an important job.

That's when I finally had to admit I needed to fix this now. I decided I needed to fully commit to fixing this problem and apply myself one hundred percent. I couldn't keep living like this. I knew there was a better life out there and I was determined to overcome sleep apnea once and for all.

And that's why you're here, too.

You've very likely had a recent wake-up call that inspired you to get this book. Maybe you've fallen asleep during important meetings at work, missed deadlines, or made mistakes that could get you in trouble. Maybe being so tired has made you grouchy with your kids, making you snap at them. Or you might be so worn out by the end of the day that you have no energy for your partner, causing tension and problems in your marriage.

These wake-up calls look different for each of us, but they all point to the same truth—sleep apnea is messing up your life and you can't ignore it anymore. The consequences are too high. Your work, your role as a parent, your relationship with your spouse, your fulfillment in life—all these important things are being affected bit by bit because of your constant tiredness.

But it's not just about strained relationships and lost productivity, sleep apnea is also hurting your physical health. Not getting enough sleep puts a lot of stress on your body, causing inflammation and weakening your immune system. Over time, this can lead to serious health problems like heart disease, high blood pressure, diabetes, and even memory loss. You may not feel the full impact yet, but make no mistake: untreated sleep apnea is a ticking time bomb for your health. The statistics are startling:

- After age 40, sleep apnea can lead to you dying 10 to 25 years earlier.
- **105 people die every single day** from sleep apnea in the United States alone.[1]
  - ◦ 33 die from a heart attack.
  - ◦ 11 die from a stroke.
  - ◦ 25 die from other problems related to sleep apnea (diabetes, cancer, crashing a car while sleepy, etc.).
  - ◦ And, 36 are found dead in bed because they suffocated while sleeping.

And I wouldn't be doing my job unless I also told you that using a CPAP does not save you from the risks of dying young like we've been told. That's what was found in a 2017 study that included data from ten trials involving 7,266 patients with sleep apnea. What they found was that using CPAP was **not linked** to reduced risk of dying from heart attacks and stroke.[2]

1 Marshall NS et al. Sleep apnea and 20-year follow-up for all-cause mortality, stroke, and cancer incidence in the Busselton Health Study cohort. J Clin Sleep Med. 2014;10(4):355-362.

2 Yu J et al. Association of Positive Airway Pressure With Cardiovascular Events and Death in Adults With Sleep Apnea: A Systematic Review and Meta-analysis. JAMA. 2017 July 11;318(2):156-166.

For the sake of the remaining years and quality of your life, that's why you're taking decisive action to fix this. So, here's how we're going to get back to sleeping quietly and waking up refreshed:

In chapter two, we're going to help you understand the root cause of obstructive sleep apnea.

In chapter three, we're going to cover why so many of the standard treatment options for sleep apnea keep you stuck.

In chapter four, we will talk about our 5-factor model for overcoming sleep apnea.

In chapter five, we're going to review the fundamental breathing routines to help you start sleeping easier as soon as tonight.

In chapter six, we will discuss the top diet hacks to make your breathing more efficient.

In chapter seven, we will talk about how to set your body's internal rhythm so that your breathing is steadier at night.

In chapter eight, we will talk about how to easily release stress for more relaxed breathing.

In chapter nine, we'll go over the fundamental environmental upgrades you can make to your bedroom for easier breathing.

In chapter ten, we will discuss how to build on these foundations and accelerate your recovery.

So, let's begin, shall we?

Time To Reflect: What's Your Wake-Up Call?

Whenever someone signs up as a client, we ask them why they decided that **now** is the time to take charge of their health and overcome sleep apnea.

Here are a few things they've shared:

"My wife was constantly worried about my loud snoring and frequent pauses in breathing at night. I knew it was affecting both our lives, and I needed to take action for the sake of our future together."

— **Robert, 55, San Diego, CA**

"I was tired of feeling tired. I missed out on so much of my life because I was always too exhausted to participate. It was time to reclaim my energy and my life."

— **Sarah, 47, Chicago, IL**

"After years of struggling with poor sleep, I finally decided enough was enough. I wanted to ensure my golden years were truly golden, not overshadowed by sleep apnea."

— **John, 70, Orlando, FL**

"At 68, I realized that my health wasn't going to improve on its own. My grandchildren deserve a more energetic grandparent, and I deserve to enjoy my retirement without being constantly fatigued."

— **Barbara, 68, Phoenix, AZ**

Dylan Petkus

Take a moment to reflect on why you've decided that now is the time to take charge of your health. Use these prompts to guide your journaling, focusing on both the negative and positive contributors to your decision.

Negative Contributors:

1. Current Challenges:
- What are the most significant health challenges you're facing right now?
- How have these challenges impacted your daily life and well-being?

2. Consequences of Inaction:
- What are the potential long-term consequences if you don't address your sleep apnea now?
- How does the thought of continuing to struggle with these issues make you feel?

Positive Contributors:

1. Goals and Aspirations:
- What health goals do you hope to achieve by addressing your sleep apnea?
- How do you envision your life improving once you've taken control of your health?

2. Motivations:
- Who or what inspires you to make this change now?
- How will improving your health benefit those around you?

Your Next Steps

Reflecting on your "why now" can provide powerful motivation as you embark on your journey to better health. Take the time to write down your thoughts, and revisit them whenever you need a reminder of why you started this journey.

Chapter 2
How You Got Here

"We can't solve problems by using the same kind of thinking we used when we created them. Doing the same thing over and over again and expecting different results is insanity. If we want different results, we have to start thinking and acting differently."
- Albert Einstein

When I first got my diagnosis, I was shocked and felt helpless. I felt even more powerless when the "only options" were a CPAP or surgery. However, I decided to take a step back and understand more about sleep apnea so I could draw my own conclusions. So, let's do the same here, shall we?

Back in the early 1900s (way before sleep studies existed), they "discovered" sleep apnea. And, in true early 1900s form, doctors would observe you in your bedroom by candlelight. So, if you think sleep studies now are a pain in the butt, be grateful you don't have someone staring at you in your own bedroom. What they observed was that people would breathe heavier, louder, and faster until they stopped breathing altogether.[3]

As they continued to investigate, they discovered a key mechanism. In 1953, Leonard Peltier MD, PhD discovered that fast breathing at night caused pauses in breathing. Moreover, it was during the inhale that this pause in breathing happened.[4] This was a huge discovery as to what caused sleep apnea. Here's a diagram to show you how sleep apnea happens:

3   Peters, B., Guilleminault, C. (2015). A Short History of Obstructive Sleep Apnea Syndrome. In: Chokroverty, S., Billiard, M. (eds) Sleep Medicine. Springer, New York, NY.

4   Peltier LF. Obstructive apnea in artificially hyperventilated subjects during sleep. J Appl Physiol. 1953 Apr;5(10):614-8

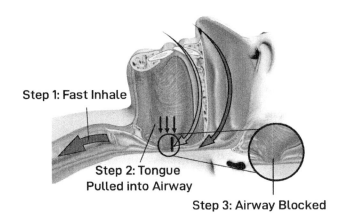

Step 1: Fast Inhale

Step 2: Tongue
Pulled into Airway

Step 3: Airway Blocked

Figure 2-3: Mechanism of obstructive sleep apnea

The reason this happens is pretty simple. Obstructive sleep apnea almost always involves something that narrows the airway. It could be your weight, an enlarged tongue, a blocked nasal passageway, etc. Regardless, all these lead to a narrow airway. ***But this narrow airway is not the only whole problem!***

The real problem starts with how our bodies compensate for this narrow airway. Now, your body still needs the same amount of air. So, your body starts to breathe faster—just like if you had to breathe through a straw.

As a result of this faster inhale, your airway will collapse, and this blocks your breathing. Think of how a paper straw can collapse when you're trying to drink a thick milkshake. The increase in suction force pulls the walls together.

Smart Cookie Question: "How is the problem breathing too fast? I thought the problem was not breathing at night?"

This is a great question, and one I'm often asked by new clients. It seems counterintuitive because we're only told about the pause in breathing (known as an apnea). However, this pause in breathing is just an effect of the main driving force (the faster inhale).

In fact, this is exactly what they found in a research study that investigated breathing very closely in sleep apnea patients.[5] They found that people with sleep apnea breathe three times faster at night than people without sleep apnea! They also noticed that the breathing got faster just before the pause in breathing.

---

5 Kwon OE et al. Tidal volume and stroke volume changes caused by respiratory events during sleep and their relationship with OSA severity: a pilot study. Sleep Breath. 2021 Dec;25(4):2025-2038

The Bottom Line

The common root cause of obstructive sleep apnea is this faster nighttime breathing. Yes, a narrow airway contributes to faster breathing. But ultimately, the main issue is faster breathing.

And this also explains the gradual onset of sleep apnea that you've experienced. If you have a true airway narrowing, it's just "there." For example, if your tongue is too big, it does not continue to get bigger over the years. However, the snoring, fatigue, and poor sleep does get worse over time.

That's why you may not have noticed the faster breathing itself, but you probably felt the effects. Gradually, you started to feel more tired in the morning as your days became harder to get through. But then, there came a point where the entire day became a struggle. The fast breathing can progress to a point where you're waking up with a pounding chest.

How Can You Confirm You Breathe Too Fast?

It's really simple and you can do this right now. In the research, this faster breathing is known as **high**

respiratory loop gain.[6] Now, that term is really catchy and approachable (I'm joking, it's horrid), which is why I mainly refer to it as plain-old faster breathing. One of the best ways to measure this is with a simple breath hold exercise that I like to call the "relaxed pause." We'll go more in depth on this in later chapters. The most important thing for you to know now is that a shorter relaxed pause means you have faster breathing. Let's go ahead and confirm if you breathe too fast by measuring your relaxed pause together.

Here's How to Measure It:

1. Sit Comfortably:
- Find a comfortable, upright sitting position where you can relax.

2. Breathe Normally:
- Take a few moments to breathe normally, allowing your breathing to settle into a natural rhythm.

3. Exhale and Hold:
- After a normal exhale, gently hold your breath. Do not forcefully inhale or exhale before holding your breath.

---

6 Messineo L et al. Breath-holding as a means to estimate the loop gain contribution to obstructive sleep apnoea. J Physiol. 2018 Sep;596(17):4043-4056.

4. Count the Seconds:

- Count how many seconds you can hold your breath comfortably before you feel the first urge to breathe (this should be a subtle feeling, not holding onto your breath for dear life).

5. Record Your Time:

- Note the number of seconds you held your breath. This is your "relaxed pause."

What Does Your Time Mean?

The more of a "fast breather" you are, then the shorter your relaxed pause will be. When I first started out, I measured 7 to 9 seconds on my first few attempts.

It is highly likely that you're less than 15 seconds, which—I will be blunt—is bad. Our first goal with our clients is to get them to 30 seconds and then 45 seconds. Again, we'll take a deeper dive into this over the next few chapters. But, before we get there, I want to show you how this real root issue explains how many traditional treatments fail us.

Smart Cookie Question:

"If a narrow airway leads to faster breathing, why not just widen the airway?"

This is one of the most common questions from clients when I explain how sleep apnea happens. And it is a good question because the sequence of events in sleep apnea is:

1. A narrowing of the airway
2. Faster breathing
3. Airway collapse

So, we should just address factor 1, right?

If we widened the airway with surgery, then the issue should be gone one hundred percent of the time, right?

Well, according to a 2020 study from Stanford, surgeries for sleep apnea only reduce the severity of sleep apnea less than half the time (43.2 percent)![7] My experience with clients backs this up, we have many people who have had various surgeries but are still struggling to breathe at night.

So, even though anatomy may have started the problem, addressing it with surgery does not fix the

---

7   Liu SY et al. Surgical Algorithm for Obstructive Sleep Apnea: An Update. Clin Exp Otorhinolaryngol. 2020 Aug;13(3):215-224.

problem. That's because the faster breathing pattern is still present, and this leads to the airway collapse at night. Once you form a bad breathing pattern, it takes time and effort to reprogram it (and that's exactly what our goal is).

Instead of working *against* your anatomy with forced air, plastic, and surgeries, we teach you how to work *with* your anatomy by focusing on the real core issue of faster nighttime breathing.

Why Don't Other Doctors Talk About This?

A lot of people are a bit shocked that their sleep doctor hasn't mentioned this. However, I'm not surprised one bit. You see, modern medicine exists with the double-edge of insurance. Yes, insurance is great for when life happens, but less so for chronic issues.

Insurance has become a naughty little secret embedded in the decision-making of physicians around the world. It is pretty common that a medication or surgery will ONLY happen if insurance will cover it. Now, I'm somewhat upset that I live in a world where a spreadsheet in an office is dictating medical care instead of a doctor.

But it actually gets worse than that. If insurance dictates treatment, it also dictates what doctors learn. Medical schools focus on treatments that are covered by insurance because that's what doctors will use in their practice. This means that if a treatment isn't covered by insurance, doctors might not learn about it at all.

In the case of sleep apnea, doctors are taught that CPAP machines are the only way. That happens because that's what insurance companies are willing to pay for. As a result, the deeper mechanisms of sleep apnea (i.e., a fast inhale) are not covered in training.

And the reason insurance companies are willing to pay for a CPAP is because that's been the only solution since the 1980s. Before then, they would just cut a hole in your throat to breathe. As you can see, the CPAP didn't have a high standard to beat.

Modern medicine went down this road because initially they couldn't find a way to slow down the breathing. So, instead, they worked around it with brute force (surgeries and CPAPs).

It's a frustrating reality. That is why it's so important to seek out information and solutions beyond the traditional medical system. By understanding the true causes of sleep apnea and exploring all available treatments, you can find a path to better sleep and better health that might not be mentioned in a typical doctor's visit.

How This All Relates To Snoring

If snoring is a big problem for you, you need to understand that snoring is a gateway to sleep apnea.

It's simple, sleep apnea is when your airway gets *completely* blocked off and snoring is your airway *almost* blocked off.

This is why 95 percent of people with sleep apnea snore. So, if you have snoring but not the traditional sleep apnea symptoms, then just know that snoring is one of the first signs of developing full blown sleep apnea.

Now, how exactly snoring happens is something I call the "whistle effect" as explained below:

1. The Whistle Effect: Imagine blowing air through a whistle. When air moves quickly through the narrow space of the whistle, it creates a loud sound. This is because the rapid airflow causes vibrations in the whistle.

2. Narrowed Airway: Similarly, in sleep apnea, the airway becomes partially blocked or narrowed during sleep. When you inhale quickly, the fast-moving air must squeeze through this tight space.

3. Vibrations Create Noise: Just like the whistle, the narrowed airway causes the tissues in your throat to vibrate as the fast-moving air passes through. These vibrations produce the sound we recognize as snoring.

4. Fast Inhale: A faster inhale increases the speed of the air passing through the constricted airway, amplifying the vibrations and making the snoring louder and more pronounced.

Understanding snoring as the "whistle effect" helps illustrate how the combination of a narrowed airway and rapid airflow can lead to the noisy disruptions characteristic of obstructive sleep apnea.

Chapter 3
Why You've Been Stuck With Sleep Apnea

There is a condition related to all diseases that Harvard, Yale, Stanford, and all those prestigious universities haven't yet caught up to. In fact, I'll go ahead and say I've discovered this condition. This condition is called "One-thing-itis." If we look in the Dylan Petkus Dictionary of Medicine (which is set to be published in 3023), then we'll read that one-thing-itis is defined as:

The hope that a health issue can be addressed by one thing. However, when one thing doesn't work, the search for another thing begins. Then, when that fails, another thing is sought out.

Now, let me confess. I would have loved a simple solution to my sleep apnea back then. But instead, I was heavily infected with one-thing-itis, and it sounded like this:

- *"Maybe this third mouth guard will work."*
- *"If the mouth guards didn't work, maybe I should try an oral appliance."*
- *"If this CPAP mask isn't working, then maybe I should try out another one."*
- *"If this pillow isn't working, maybe I should try this other, fluffier one."*
- *"Oh, mouth tape looks cool! Let me try that!"*

Don't get me wrong, if you have one-thing-itis (like I did), it means you're putting in a great effort. But you just need to direct that effort toward a more comprehensive system that works (and we'll get to that soon!).

When you have one-thing-itis, every step takes you further away from the core issue at hand. As a result, there is a ton of wasted time, money, and effort. But worst of all is the defeat you feel. Every failed attempt chips away at your hope, leaving you feeling more and more helpless. You start to doubt if you'll ever find relief, and the frustration and despair can become overwhelming.

You might feel like giving up, thinking that nothing will ever work for you. This emotional toll is exhausting and can make the journey to finding a real solution feel even more daunting.

You're already one step closer to curing one-thing-itis by understanding the core of sleep apnea. Now, we have to make sure you understand why so many things have failed you in the past. That way, we can pull out the "weeds" before starting to plant some new truths.

The CPAP Machine: A Nightly Hassle

CPAP (Continuous Positive Airway Pressure) therapy is widely recommended for treating obstructive sleep apnea, but let's face it, using a CPAP machine can feel like a nightmare, with a mask strapped to your face and a tube rolling around in the bed with you. The mask can cause nasal congestion, dryness, and even inflammation.[8] Many users report waking up with a dry mouth or a stuffy nose, making it even harder to breathe comfortably throughout the night.

Then there's the psychological impact. The constant noise of the CPAP machine and the feeling of being tethered to it can severely disturb not just your sleep but also your partner's. Imagine trying to rest with a machine

---

8 Koutsourelakis I et al. Nasal inflammation in sleep apnoea patients using CPAP and effect of heated humidification. Eur Respir J. 2011 Mar;37(3):587-94.

humming next to you all night, or the disruption from your partner adjusting their mask repeatedly. This constant disturbance can lead to significant sleep deprivation for both individuals. Over time, the frustration and exhaustion from these nightly disruptions can strain the relationship, leading to emotional stress and resentment. Many partners dread going to bed, knowing they face another night of disrupted sleep, which can erode intimacy and negatively impact their overall quality of life.

Moreover, CPAP machines are not cheap. A CPAP usually costs between $500 and $1,000, and insurance doesn't always cover the full cost. Then, there is the cost of all the accessories you have to replace—unless you want to deal with lung and throat infections. Here's the breakdown for the maintenance costs:

Accessory	Per Item	Replacements Per Year	Annual Cost
Masks	$50 - $200	4	$200 - $800
Headgear	$15 - $40	2	$30 - $80
Tubing	$10 - $50	2	$20 - $100
Filters	$4 - $20	4	$16 - $80
Humidifier	$15 - $40	2	$30 - $80
Cleaning supplies	$80 - $200	1	$80 - $200

Table 3-1: CPAP annual maintenance and costs

So, let's assume you live in a perfect world where your insurance covers your CPAP (good luck), using a CPAP will cost you $376 to $1,340 per year.

Dependency on the device is another concern. Many users find they can't sleep without their CPAP once they've started using it. Any interruption in using the machine, like during travel or power outages, can immediately bring back sleep apnea symptoms.

That's what makes a CPAP a crutch. Now, crutches are great temporary aids when you break a bone, but long-term they cause soreness and strain. That's how I view CPAPs, as a short-term aid but not a lasting solution (and the inventor of the CPAP agrees with me, more on that below).

And, just like a band-aid for someone who needs surgery, the underlying issues continue to get worse which **leads us to the "dirty little secret" of CPAP.** A 2017 study from the Journal of the American Medical Association[9] (one of the biggest journals in medicine) found that using a CPAP was not associated with a decrease in deaths from heart attack and all other causes of death. In other words, **CPAP therapy does not extend your lifespan.**

---

9   Yu Jet al. Association of Positive Airway Pressure With Cardiovascular Events and Death in Adults With Sleep Apnea: A Systematic Review and Meta-analysis. JAMA. 2017 July 11;318(2):156-166.

I believe the reason for this lackluster effect is that CPAPs prevent you from achieving optimal sleep. When you don't have one hundred percent natural sleep, then your body is not able to fully restore itself. Then, as a result, diseases continue to progress that shave years off your life.

If CPAP didn't "work" for you, it is not your fault!

Now, there may be some people who love their CPAP who read this book. And, if your CPAP works for you and you're happy as a clam, then that's great!

However, if you're a part of the 70 percent of people who can't get CPAP to work,[10] I want you to know it's not your fault! Don't let people guilt trip you for not putting up with the hassle of the CPAP at night. It's not because of your willpower or effort.

A CPAP may be considered the "gold standard" in sleep apnea care today, but it is really just "the best option" modern medicine has. Still, it is a step up from putting a hole in peoples' throats, which was the go-to care throughout the 1950s and into the 1970s. Seriously, the "gold standard" for sleep apnea

---

10 Qiao M et al. Long term adherence to continuous positive Airway pressure in mild obstructive sleep apnea. BMC Pulm Med. 2023 Sep 1;23(1):320

Dylan Petkus

treatment used to be a tracheostomy, after which you breathed through a hole in your throat. A CPAP is definitely better than that, but don't settle for an option that can cause more harm than good (e.g., the 2023 recalls on CPAPs causing lung cancer).

In fact, one of the inventors of the CPAP, Colin Sullivan, has been quoted saying, *"CPAPs were always intended to be a temporary physical therapy measure, not a permanent solution."*[11]

Another big concern is what CPAP manufacturers are hiding from us. I say this not as a conspiracy theory but based on recent events in the CPAP industry. Philips Respironics recently reached a $1.1 billion settlement over CPAP lawsuits, acknowledging the severe health risks posed by their devices. This massive settlement includes $1.075 billion set aside to compensate patients who suffered serious injuries or complications (**such as cancer**) from using recalled Philips CPAP machines, and an additional $25 million for medical monitoring of those at risk.

Lastly, as with band-aids, a CPAP also does nothing to fix the real problem (faster breathing). This has been known since 1985 when they studied whether the fast breathing (known as "daytime loop gain" in the research literature) changed after giving patients CPAP treatment.

11 Rozsa, M. (2023, October 23). The inventor of the CPAP machine wishes for a future where his device is no longer needed. Salon

Results showed there was no change in the breathing pattern for these patients.[12] The reason for this is obvious: a CPAP "breathes for you" and does not correct the real breathing problem. This is a theme you'll see with all the other band-aid solutions including the next one: mouth guards.

Mouth Guards: Painful and Temporary

Mouth guards (we'll also include oral appliances, mandibular advancement devices, etc. in this category), often prescribed for sleep apnea, are fundamentally a band-aid solution. They work by adding a few more centimeters of space in the airway opening, which can temporarily reduce apnea episodes. However, as the underlying breathing issue continues to get worse, these few extra centimeters aren't enough to keep your airway open. That's why so many people must constantly adjust their mouth guards or try new ones!

Another concern is the fragility of mouth guards. A mouth guard only works **if it stays in your mouth.** I know for myself and many of our clients, this is a struggle for them. They wake up groggy and exhausted to see their mouth guard beside their pillow. So, once again, we

12 Deacon-Diaz NL et al. Daytime loop gain is elevated in obstructive sleep apnea but not reduced by CPAP treatment. J Appl Physiol (1985). 2018 Nov 1;125(5):1490-1497.

have a temporary fix that does little to improve long-term health and can lull patients into a false sense of security, thinking they are treating their condition when they are merely masking it.

Moreover, the use of mouthguards can lead to significant and irreversible dental issues. Prolonged use often results in jaw pain, bite changes, and tooth movement, creating new health problems while trying to mitigate another. A study in the Journal of Dental Sleep Medicine reports that about 30 percent of mouth guard users experience adverse effects such as these.[13] These dental changes can require further treatment, adding to the physical and financial burden on patients. And that is on top of the three to four annual replacements for a mouth guard that can run from $100 to $150 (a grand total of $300 to $600 per year on mouth plastic). And, if you go for a fancy oral appliance from your dentist, that can range from $1,000 to $4,000. That's a steep price for never fixing the real issue.

Mouth Tape: Trendy but Ineffective

Mouth tape, a trendy solution for sleep apnea, is literally and figuratively a band-aid that fails to address the

13 Sheats, R. D. (2020). Management of side effects of oral appliance therapy for sleep-disordered breathing: Summary of American Academy of Dental Sleep Medicine recommendations. Journal of Clinical Sleep Medicine 16(5), 835.

underlying issues of the condition. The idea behind mouth tape is to force nasal breathing by taping the mouth shut. However, this completely ignores the underlying reason as to why people are breathing through their mouth in the first place.

Mouth breathing happens because of faster breathing. Think of your nose as a narrow straw and your mouth as a wide straw. When you breathe slowly, the narrow straw (your nose) works just fine, allowing enough air to pass through comfortably. However, when you start breathing faster, the narrow straw can't handle the increased airflow demand. At this point, your body instinctively opens the wide straw (your mouth) to allow more air in.

Faster breathing increases the airflow demand, and since your nose has a limit to how much air it can handle, it reaches its maximum capacity. When this happens, the resistance in your nasal passages forces your mouth to open to compensate and provide enough air, leading to mouth breathing. Thus, just taping your mouth will not fix the problem. In fact, mouth taping is just like wagging your dog's tail in the hopes you'll make him happy.

Now, there is research to suggest mouth taping can help with very mild cases of sleep apnea. One study looked at the effect of mouth taping on AHI (Apnea Hypopnea Index), which is the main number on your sleep study they'll give you. The results were underwhelming as the

AHI went from 8.3 to 4.7.[14] Now, these were patients with very mild sleep apnea. At present, there is no research to suggest that people with moderate to severe sleep apnea benefit from mouth taping. That's why many of my clients report mouth tape as something that made no difference for them in the past.

Furthermore, using mouth tape can pose significant risks and discomfort. Many users experience skin irritation, allergic reactions, or a sense of panic and claustrophobia from having their mouths taped shut. There are also safety concerns, especially for individuals who have nasal obstructions or conditions like a deviated septum, which can make nasal breathing difficult or impossible. The lack of reliable adhesion can also lead to the tape coming off during the night, making it an unreliable option. Collectively, these factors make mouth tape a dubious and fragile solution.

Surgery: Irreversible and Risky

With the hyper-focus on anatomy, surgery sounds like a decent option. Sure, you'll have a hard recovery period, but the problem should be gone because the only issue is anatomy, right?

14 Lee YC et al. The Impact of Mouth-Taping in Mouth-Breathers with Mild Obstructive Sleep Apnea: A Preliminary Study. Healthcare (Basel). 2022 Sep 13;10(9):1755

Well, when you have a half-truth for the problem, you achieve half-results. That's why a review in the Journal of Otolaryngology-Head & Neck Surgery done by Stanford University found that the surgical success rate for sleep apnea is 43.2 percent, with many patients experiencing a return of symptoms over time.[15] I don't know about you, but I don't like to gamble with my health.

To further back up my theory of faster breathing being the biggest issue, "non-responders" to surgery can be predicted by just how bad their breathing is. One study found that patients with higher "respiratory loop gain" (the scientific way of saying "fast breathing at night") were more likely to **not** benefit from surgery.[16]

So, once more, it is clear the major contributor to sleep apnea is faster breathing. Fortunately, fixing your breathing is a lot easier than surgery.

Inspire Therapy:
A Shocking New Option

If you're like me and get a lot of ads while on social media, you may have heard about the Inspire surgery.

15 Liu SY, Riley RW, Yu MS. Surgical Algorithm for Obstructive Sleep Apnea: An Update. Clin Exp Otorhinolaryngol. 2020 Aug;13(3):215-224

16 Joosten SA et al. Loop Gain Predicts the Response to Upper Airway Surgery in Patients With Obstructive Sleep Apnea. Sleep. 2017 Jul 1;40(7)

Dylan Petkus

It sounds great at first! All you do is click a button and then technology works its magic to stimulate your airway muscles. To achieve that, you only have to get an electronic device implanted in your chest wall. But don't forget the wire they have to run through your neck and into your throat muscles. Oh, and then you'll need to wait a month or two as the scars heal before you can "activate your device."

Once you activate your device, it's smooth sailing, right? Obviously, the answer is a resounding 'no' (just in case you haven't detected my sarcasm yet).

After all that, then you'll have to work alongside your surgeon's team to get the right amount of electroshock to your airway muscles and tongue at night. This only takes three to twelve months to get right! If you don't get woken up by the electrostimulation, then you might get some decent sleep. And, if you miss seeing your surgeon after a few years, don't worry! That's because you will have to undergo periodic surgical revisions along the way.

Now, don't get me wrong. I'm not saying the Inspire works for no one. I'm saying that their marketing team has done a top-notch job at making surgery and implanting medical devices look as simple as turning on a TV with a remote.

Let's have an honest conversation about the Inspire. First, if you'd like, you can go to their Facebook groups, where you'll notice something rather interesting. This will require you to sit and refresh the posts in the group every twenty minutes, but it's worth it (to me at least). At first you'll notice a lot of support for the Inspire (again, it does work for some people). But, the moment you see a negative post describing complications or regrets about getting the device, that post will disappear in about twenty minutes to two hours. (If it sounds like I sit on my computer all day, rest assured, I do.)

This reflects exactly what we see in research literature, too. Now, I'll give Inspire credit as they share their research results. And you'll see great statistics that make you excited about this device. However, most people don't click to read the studies. And most people don't buy the actual studies and then comb through the results (I'm a statistics snob and proud of it).

But if you did, you'd discover that these studies often use something known as a "sub-group analysis." This is when you only look at certain parts of the data set. For instance, let's say I eat well Monday through Friday, but on Saturday and Sunday I sit on the couch and eat twinkies. Overall, my diet would be average. However, if I did a sub-group analysis where I ignored Saturday and Sunday, then I'm a very healthy eater. But is that really the truth? Obviously not. Those days of unhealthy eating can't be ignored.

The sub-group analyses show that half of people don't respond favorably to Inspire (and similar) surgeries. That is a whopping fifty percent of people who get ignored. And they get ignored because if you include them, then Inspire only provides a thirty percent improvement in symptoms. If you ignore those pesky non-responders, Inspire provides a sixty percent improvement.[17] Which statistic do you think sells more surgeries?

Again, my only goal here is to give you a realistic picture of the options so that you can make better decisions. That's why I encourage you to move beyond the band-aids so you can address the real problems with fewer risks and side effects.

Moving Beyond Band-Aids

That's why we're going to dive even deeper into this fast breathing at night and discuss how to comprehensively address it in the next chapter.

Get Your Sleep Apnea Score

To help you get a crystal-clear understanding of where you stand with sleep apnea, I wanted to offer an assessment we use exclusively with our clients. It is a quick, researched-backed assessment that helps you identify several factors.

---

17 Costantino A et al. Hypoglossal nerve stimulation long-term clinical outcomes: a systematic review and meta-analysis. Sleep Breath. 2020 Jun;24(2):399-411

- **The Relaxed Pause:** I provide a video to make sure you measure this critical metric correctly.
- **Sleepiness Severity:** Discover how your sleep apnea impacts your daily energy levels and overall alertness.
- **Quality of Life:** Gain a comprehensive understanding of how sleep apnea may be influencing your overall well-being.
- **Longevity:** Understand the potential impact of sleep apnea on your lifespan.

Ultimately, you'll get a **Sleep Apnea Severity Score** that makes it easy to identify where you are and help you track progress along your journey. Go ahead and take a few minutes to fill this out and get your results instantly:

TheSleepApneaSolution.com/score

Or, even if you're not a tech-person, you can use your phone's camera to focus on the code below, and then touch the link that pops up on your phone to navigate to the assessment.

Chapter 4
Breathing Your Way To Better Sleep

We're going to do a high-level overview of how you fix the root issue of sleep apnea (a faster inhale). Then, in each specific chapter, we'll go a bit deeper into the details of how these factors work.

At a high level, sleep apnea happens because of fast breathing that pulls your airway shut (I think I have mentioned this a few times). Thus, to fix sleep apnea, you just need to slow down your breathing at night. Then, as shown in Figure 4-4, your tongue stays out of your airway, and you can breathe more easily at night.

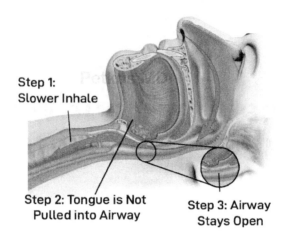

Step 1:
Slower Inhale

Step 2: Tongue is Not
Pulled into Airway

Step 3: Airway
Stays Open

Figure 4-4: Airway physiology without fast breathing

So, all we have to do is slow down your breathing. The best way to directly impact breathing is with the breathing routines (chapter 5). But, just like a bad infomercial— *"but wait, there's more!"*—there are other ways to indirectly improve breathing as I discovered along my journey (chapters 6 through 9).

There are five factors in total. And, in what might be the greatest achievement of my life, they all fit into a neat little acronym of S.L.E.E.P.

Here are the five factors of the S.L.E.E.P. model:

1. **S**low Breathing
2. **L**ower Stress
3. **E**stablish Rhythm
4. **E**nhance Environment
5. **P**rioritize Nutrition

Let's continue my journey from the first chapter to discuss how this was all uncovered.

Slow Breathing

The first factor in fixing sleep apnea is what led me on this journey. As we both know, one of the biggest issues with sleep apnea is how we breathe at night.

This is due to anatomical issues that alter something known as the **Brain-Breath Connection**. This concept is simple and intuitive. For instance, if you focus on slower breathing, what happens to your breathing after you stop focusing on it? It continues to be slow and steady. Conversely, if you breathe rapidly, what happens when you stop focusing on it? It remains fast. This connection illustrates how your brain and breathing muscles collaborate to regulate your breathing when you're not consciously controlling it.

When your airway narrows, **you must breathe faster to obtain the same amount of air**, which leads to faster-than-normal breathing when you can't focus on it, like at night. Remember, breathing too fast at night can cause airway collapse.

This understanding helped me realize why the first factor of the S.L.E.E.P. method is to "slow your breathing." By consciously practicing slower, more relaxed breathing during the day, we can reprogram our brain-breath connection to maintain a steadier and more open airway at night. This simple yet powerful technique helps minimize the occurrence of sleep apnea episodes and promotes more restful, restorative sleep.

Smart Cookie Question: "I can't control my breathing at night, how is this going to even work?"

At first glance, the connection between doing breathing exercises, lifestyle changes, and environmental fixes with breathing at night doesn't make sense.

After all, the other approaches have us strapped to a machine or with a mouth guard in our mouth all night, so how do these daytime activities work at night?

The answer is what we just talked about with the **brain-breath** connection. When you directly work on your breathing (with the breathing exercises) and indirectly work on your breathing (through lowering stress, improving nutrition, enhancing your environment, and establishing a good circadian rhythm), then this will all work together to "set" your breathing to "slower" at nighttime.

This happens because you form a better "muscle memory" with your breathing patterns that carries over into the night. Thus, your efforts during the day work on autopilot for you at night. As a result, you breathe more slowly, keep your airway open, snore less, and wake up more refreshed.

My personal journey began with trying breathing exercises to slow down my breathing. Initially, I was skeptical. In all honesty, I thought this was the dumbest thing I've tried yet. That's because everything I read suggested I needed a CPAP, surgery, or some device in my mouth.

However, I was shocked when I woke up the next morning without waking up once for the first time in months. Seriously, I was so shocked I thought it was more likely that someone drugged me earlier that day than breathing exercises helped my sleep. I was absolutely floored.

I felt like I had unlocked the secrets of the universe. I felt pretty smug, thinking, "I got it!" However, life would humble me as the effectiveness of the breathing exercises faded with time. That's what led me to 1) panic a bit and 2) discover the next factor.

Lowering Stress

As my journey continued, I realized the importance of the next factor due to my constant feelings of being on edge throughout the day. I was overwhelmed by work and irritable with everyone around me. This is because sleep apnea puts our nervous system in overdrive. An overactive nervous system worsens breathing issues by causing faster breathing and a lack of muscle tone in the airway. So, to *indirectly help with breathing*, all I had to do was lower my stress.

However, I was unable to quit my job and move to a secluded island with 5-star amenities (maybe you can relate). I had to think of how to better deal with stress instead of fully getting rid of it. So, I developed efficient and powerful practices to lower my stress levels without putting my life on hold. Once I implemented these practices, I noticed a steadier mood during the day and deeper sleep at night.

This was a big milestone for me because I realized something not directly tied to my breathing could affect my breathing, even at a later time. You see, our bodies are complex, which is bad when trying to fix them, but it is great when we find new ways to address our problems. This motivated my search for other factors that targeted the core issue of fast breathing. As I began to feel more in control and less stressed, I realized there was another crucial element to address: the rhythm of my daily routine.

Dylan Petkus

Establishing Your Rhythm

Next, I noticed how quickly my sleep schedule could go off track. One bad night would lead to early bedtimes, naps during the day, and a vicious cycle that worsened my sleep apnea. I learned that our body's rhythm impacts our breathing and that disrupting this rhythm increases episodes of gasping or pauses in breathing.

I figured out which factors (lighting, bedtime, etc.) were most important to establish a healthy rhythm. This led to easier breathing, deeper sleep, and fewer nighttime awakenings. It was like a flipped switch. Almost immediately, my body began to sync up with a more natural, healthy pattern.

After stabilizing my sleep schedule, I was still far from one hundred percent and would experience big swings in my sleep. That's what brought me to the next step in my journey.

Enhancing Your Environment

At one point, I was traveling frequently, and my sleep varied wildly from one place to another. I realized that environmental factors like air quality, humidity, and even scents played a significant role in my sleep apnea. Creating a sleep-friendly environment promotes clear airways and relaxation.

I addressed hundreds of possible environmental factors, and some were absolute game changers. I slept through the night and woke up feeling like a million bucks, thinking I was finally "done" with sleep apnea.

But even with a perfect environment, I noticed there were still fluctuations in my sleep quality, which led me to consider another critical factor.

Prioritizing Nutrition

I want to take a moment to pause and reflect on why nutrition is the last factor. Usually, nutrition or diet is one of the first things people think about with "lifestyle management of sleep apnea." However, it is only one factor that can impact your breathing.

And, before you spiral into diet-PTSD, let me assure you that you don't need to lose a pound to get better sleep. Now, don't get me wrong, a healthy weight is great for sleep. I'm just saying that you don't need to wait four months for weight loss to happen.

I realized nutrition was a big factor but for a different reason other than weight loss (especially because I was not overweight). Instead, I noticed that my sleep apnea symptoms fluctuated depending on what I ate. This led me to understand the importance of nutrition in maintaining clear airways and promoting restful sleep. Curious to explore this potential link, I began keeping a food diary and paying close attention to how different meals and snacks affected my sleep quality.

By experimenting with different combinations and timing of meals, I developed a clearer understanding of which nutrients and eating habits had the most positive impact on my sleep apnea symptoms. Simple, targeted adjustments to my diet led to more stable breathing and more restful sleep.

Altogether Now!

Each of these factors—slowing your breathing, lowering stress, establishing rhythm, enhancing your environment, and prioritizing nutrition—played a crucial role in my journey to overcome sleep apnea. By integrating these elements into your life, you can start to reclaim your nights and your life, one breath at a time.

Please behold the peak of my artistic skills and see how it all comes together:

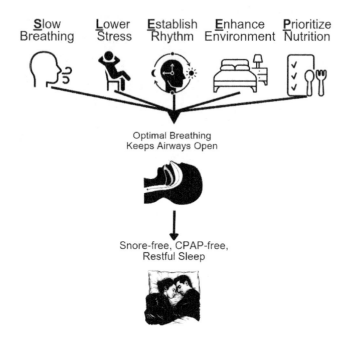

Figure 4-5: S.L.E.E.P. definition, dynamics, and results

Altogether, it took me two years of tinkering around until I had full resolution. Now, don't freak out. A lot of that was trial and error, which we're eliminating as best as we can with this book. Many of our clients are sleeping better, snoring less, and are off their CPAP within a few months.

For myself, the turnaround was huge. I awoke with energy, mental clarity, and motivation I hadn't felt in years. I could exercise, socialize, and take on big projects without collapsing. I felt in control of my life again.

Work became easy again. My mind felt sharp and focused once more. I powered through complex protocols without losing concentration. In meetings, I engaged actively in lively conversations instead of nodding off in my chair.

My social life regained its spark too. Hikes and dinners with friends became fun again instead of exhausting chores. I felt fully aligned—the person everyone saw on the outside was aligned with who I truly was on the inside. I no longer had to put on a fake smile.

Most importantly, I no longer thought about my health all the time, either. The constant worry faded into the background. Taking care of myself became simple and intuitive.

These victories were not just about better sleep; they were about reclaiming my life. Each day, I woke up feeling refreshed and ready to conquer whatever challenges lay ahead. No longer was I dragging through the day in a fog of exhaustion. Instead, I was living with purpose and joy.

Bottom Line:

If you were to explain to your wife, husband, or other family member what you're doing, it would be as simple as:

"I'm undoing my sleep apnea with breathing exercises, stress reduction, routines that set my body's rhythm, environmental

fixes, and nutrition upgrades, all aimed at slowing down my breathing at night so my airway stays open"

Or, even simpler, you could say *"Breathing exercises and targeted, healthy lifestyle changes help me breath better at night."*

And, if for some reason you were stuck explaining this book at a dinner party, then I have you covered:

Q: How does slower breathing even help with sleep apnea?

- *A: "Slower breathing reduces the chances of my airway collapsing during sleep, which helps me breathe easier and sleep better."*

Q: How do breathing exercises help with sleep apnea?

- *A: "Breathing exercises train my body to breathe more efficiently and calmly, especially at night, which helps keep my airway open."*

Q: How does stress reduction help with sleep apnea?

- *A: "Reducing stress lowers my overall breathing rate and prevents the rapid breathing that can cause my airway to collapse."*

Q: How do routines that set your body's rhythm help with sleep apnea?

- **A:** *"This regulates my body's internal clock, making it easier to get restful sleep and reduce sleep apnea episodes."*

Q: How do environmental fixes help with sleep apnea?

- **A:** *"Optimizing my environment promotes better sleep quality and reduces airway irritation."*

Q: How does nutrition help with sleep apnea?

- **A:** *"Improving my nutrition reduces inflammation, which helps keep my airway open and improves my breathing at night."*

And Here's The Most Important Question:

"Does this actually work?"

At the end of the day, the science can make sense, but the most important thing is real-world results. That's why I'll share client success stories throughout the book. But I also want to give you the big picture before starting out. That's why I want to share research on our clients' results with you.

Now, I want to manage some expectations before I show you this data. In terms of results from this book, I get at least one email a week that says something along the lines of:

"Thank you so much, Dr. Petkus! This book was a game changer for me!"

However, I don't have the ability to combine all the data from all the thousands of people who have gotten this book. Instead, I can only show you the data from the close work with our clients. Obviously, reading a book and working directly with us are both good, yet very different. My goal in sharing this data is to show you what is possible. As much as I wish I could, I can't guarantee that you'll get the same or better results than our clients. With that disclaimer out of the way, let's go over the data. With our clients we track a few important variables, from sleep surveys to sleep data at night.

When looking at sleep quality using the Pittsburgh Sleep Quality Index (the most commonly used survey tool in sleep research), we found a seventy-six percent improvement in sleep quality. **It is important to know that a lower score is better.**

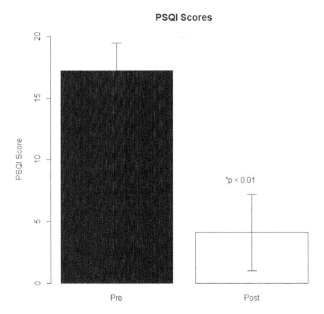

Figure 4-6: Sleep quality before and after intervention

We also used the same survey that sleep doctors use known as the Epworth Sleepiness scale. What we found is that our clients had an eighty percent reduction in daytime sleepiness as shown below:

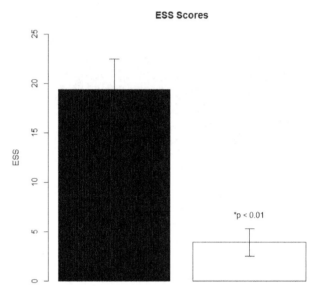

Figure 4-7: Daytime sleepiness before and after intervention

Now, if you're hoping to see more objective data, then this next graph is for you. We measured AHI which is an index of how bad sleep apnea is. A higher AHI is worse. Now, these measurements were done without the use of a CPAP. Oftentimes, clients will report the AHI from their machine, but that is a "fake" low score because the machine is basically breathing for you. With that being said, we see a roughly sixty-seven percent reduction in AHI as shown below:

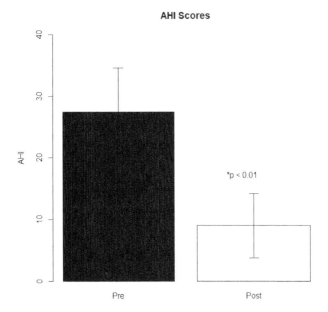

Figure 4-8: AHI before and after intervention

For clients with partners, we had them ask about their snoring. What we found was that, before working with us, ninety-one percent of partners complained about snoring. After working with us, the complaints of snoring went down to twelve percent!

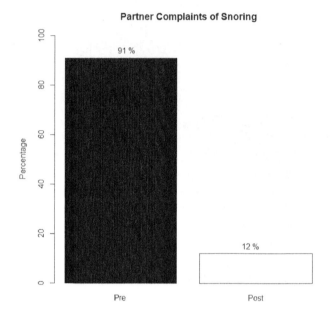

Figure 4-9: Partner complaints of snoring before and after intervention

Another common question we get from clients is, *"Can I get off this dang CPAP?"* At the beginning of our client relationships, we find that twenty-three percent of them are "CPAP-free." After we're finished working together, eighty-three percent of them are CPAP-free, as shown below:

Dylan Petkus

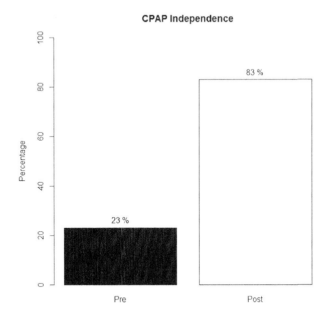

Figure 4-10: CPAP independence before and after intervention

Altogether, these results are why ninety-four percent of our clients prefer this method to CPAP and other alternatives. And ninety-one percent of them would recommend this method to someone else.

Now, I also want to be clear regarding the biggest factor for someone's success as they're about to set out on their journey. The biggest factor is how much action someone takes. We give our clients action steps every week and we monitor how they're doing with breathing exercises and lifestyle changes. It may not surprise you, but the more someone does, the faster they get to one hundred percent symptom reduction as shown below:

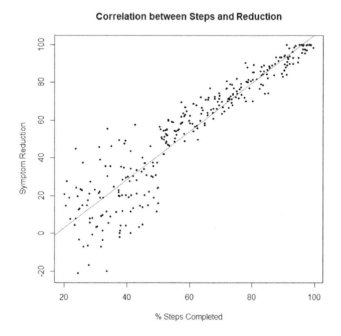

Figure 4-11: Correlation between steps completed and symptom reduction

This graph shows the relationship between the percentage of steps completed and the reduction of symptoms. Each dot represents a person who participated in the program. The line running through the dots is a trend line, showing the overall pattern of the data.

Dylan Petkus

Here Are the Key Points From Graph Above:

1. **Positive Trend**: The upward line shows that people who completed more steps generally saw more improvement in their symptoms.
2. **Some Variation**: Not everyone who did a lot of steps had the same improvement, but most did better.
3. **Takeaway**: Doing more of the program steps usually helps reduce symptoms more.

In simple terms, when you have a proven plan that yields positive outcomes, the more effort you put in, the better results you'll get out.

"But what if I have [insert anatomical issue]?"

The biggest benefit of the S.L.E.E.P. method is that this helps your body breathe with your anatomy instead of fighting against it with surgery, CPAP, mouth guards, and more.

That is what allows this method to work even if you have an enlarged tongue, big tonsils, an enlarged soft palate, a deviated septum, etc.

When your body breathes correctly, that is what will help you overcome any anatomical issue. And, if you're overweight, you don't need to lose any weight with this approach before feeling the benefits. (I'm still an advocate for a healthy weight.)

And, this method can help you no matter how severe your sleep apnea is. We've worked with clients with AHIs in the 80's and have gotten them sleeping normally again.

The Action Steps In The Book

Now, I wish there was a one-size-fits-all solution for sleep apnea. The Sleep Apnea Solution is the closest I could get.

All our clients have *different needs* despite having a *common issue*. This is why my team and I spend a lot of our time personalizing their protocols and action steps.

If I could magically know everything about you, I could write a perfect book that would 1) meet every need you have, 2) help you perfectly fit it into your lifestyle, and 3) predict future needs. As I'm updating this in 2024, that is not possible.

Nonetheless, in working with hundreds of awesome people from all walks of life, I've found many common denominators that will help most people who struggle with sleep apnea. That's what this book is.

I highlight these factors for a few reasons:

1. **Personalization is Key:** While this book provides a comprehensive guide, it's important to remember that you might need to tweak certain aspects to better suit your specific circumstances. Everyone's journey is unique, and you should feel empowered to make adjustments as needed.

2. **Manage Expectations:** It's crucial to approach this journey with realistic expectations. Some people will have the same experience I had with the breathing exercises. Others may take a bit more time and experimentation. Don't be discouraged if you don't see immediate results.

3. **See "Failure" As Feedback:** Another possibility is that some of the action steps may do diddly-squat (nothing) for you. However, that means there is likely something unique standing in the way and blocking those action steps from doing their work. This is a common issue I run into with clients, and it requires a bit of troubleshooting.

I hesitated on having this box here at all. But I wanted to have an honest conversation with you. Even though this book has great strategies, there is no silver bullet that works overnight for everyone. I wish there was.

Guess what? You're still on the fastest path to snore-free, CPAP-free, refreshing sleep. Yes, there might be some bumps along the way, but that's what makes the journey meaningful.

Embrace the process, be patient with yourself, and trust that each step brings you closer to the restful, rejuvenating sleep you deserve.

Chapter 5
Optimized Breathing

I want to address a common misconception about these breathing exercises before we dive into them. When working with one client that we'll call Mike, I asked him in his first week of working with us how important the breathing exercises were to his success. He replied with *"I'd imagine they are pretty much responsible for all my results."*

Fast forward three months later, Mike has refreshing, easy sleep and great daytime energy and I asked him the same question. This time, he gave a very calculated answer of, *"I'd say they are about thirty to forty percent."*

Mike was spot-on correct the second time. This is a typical occurrence with many of our clients. That's because we, as humans, tend to have the dreaded "one-thing-itis" I mentioned earlier. A big part of that is because modern medicine has Pill A for Disease A and Pill B for Disease B.

Instead, I encourage you to see how we're addressing sleep apnea with a holistic system that targets one specific mechanism (faster breathing at night). Yes, we are indeed doing breathing exercises to **directly impact your breathing at night.** And, yes, these breathing exercises contribute the most to your success. But, at the same time, the other four factors contribute sixty to seventy percent of your success by **indirectly impacting nighttime breathing.** This is great news because instead of depending on just one action to achieve success, multiple factors are working together for your benefit. And there are multiple levels within each of these factors that provide plenty of opportunity to improve. So, let's dive into the detail on how these exercises work.

How The Breathing Exercises Work

The breathing exercises work by directly targeting the brain-breath connection we mentioned earlier. You can think of this like "muscle memory," similar to how a person can ride a bike effortlessly after learning as a child, even after not riding for years. But instead of your leg and core muscles, your diaphragm (which is the main breathing muscle) has this muscle memory. For breathing, you can think of muscle memory as a dial that has settings from "very slow" to "very fast."

After years of breathing through a narrow airway, the muscle memory of your diaphragm gets set to "fast." So, our goal with these breathing exercises is to reset it to "slow." That way, over time, you will start to breathe slower and more steadily during both day and night. This is how breathing exercises at any time (especially before bedtime) lead to slower breathing that keeps your airways open at night.

What The Research Says About Breathing Exercises for Sleep Apnea

One study combining data from six studies involving over a thousand patients found that breathing exercises alone could reduce the number of sleep apnea events by half and can increase daytime energy by about seventy to ninety percent.[18]

Another study included a series of case studies that shared how severe sleep apnea patients were able to get off their CPAPs and be sleep apnea free based on follow up sleep studies.[19]

---

18 Cavalcante-Leão BL et al. S. Effects of respiratory training on obstructive sleep apnea: systematic review and meta-analysis. Sleep Breath. 2022 Dec;26(4):1527-1537.

19 Courtney R. Breathing retraining in sleep apnoea: a review of approaches and potential mechanisms. Sleep Breath. 2020 Dec;24(4):1315-1325.

Despite being supported in the research, this approach is not practiced widely. That is just how science and medicine work. It takes an idea about fifteen to twenty-five years to enter common knowledge and practice. However, this is much better than it used to be as it took 150 years for hand-washing to become common practice.[20]

Let's Start To Slow Down Your Breathing!

In the next few pages, we'll go over your baseline measurement, what it means, and the exercises that will help you improve. At the very end of this chapter is a link to download audio files with the exercises. That way, all you need to do is press play and follow along!

Revisiting The Relaxed Pause

Now, as you set out on your journey to improve your breathing, we need to have a way to measure your progress over time. That's what the relaxed pause is for. The relaxed pause is defined as:

How long you can comfortably hold your breath after a normal exhale.

---

20 Poczai P, Karvalics LZ. The little-known history of cleanliness and the forgotten pioneers of handwashing. Front Public Health. 2022 Oct 20;10:979464.

Dylan Petkus

More importantly, the relaxed pause is a measure of how fast you breathe at night. As you know, faster nighttime breathing pulls your tongue back to block your airway, resulting in snoring and apnea episodes.

The relationship between the relaxed pause and nighttime breathing is like a seesaw. Relaxed pause duration is on the left of the seesaw. Breathing speed (and, thus, snoring and apnea episodes) are on the right of the seesaw.

When the relaxed pause time is lower, then breathing speed is faster, snoring is louder, and apnea episodes increase.

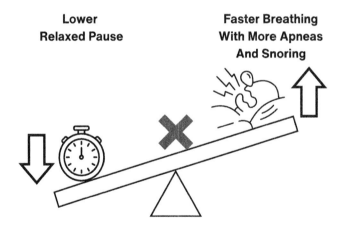

Figure 5-12: Lower relaxed pause is related to faster breathing, more apneas, and more snoring

On the other hand, when the relaxed pause time is higher, breathing speed is slower, snoring is reduced, and apnea episodes decrease.

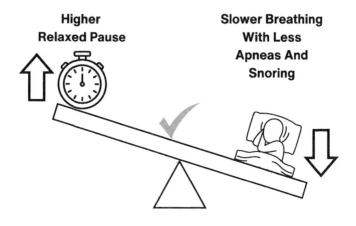

Figure 5-13: Higher relaxed pause is related to slower breathing, fewer apneas, and less snoring

Pulmonology Deep Dive
If you'd like to understand a bit more on the physiology behind the relaxed pause, this breakout box is for you. If this information is a bit dense, don't worry, the seesaw analogy explains the most important concepts. The following is for those curious about the full physiology.

The main idea is that the relaxed pause measures your body's carbon dioxide (CO_2) tolerance which reflects your breathing speed.

Here's what you need to know to make sense of that:

1. CO_2 is a byproduct of metabolism that builds up in your body until you exhale.
2. CO_2 sends a signal to your brain that tells your body to exhale.
3. How quickly your body responds to this signal is known as CO_2 tolerance. High tolerance means you need more CO_2 to send the signal to breathe. Low tolerance means you need less CO_2 to send the signal to breathe.
4. If your ***brain-breath connection*** is set to "slow," then you have higher amounts of CO_2. This means your body is more familiar with CO_2. Thus, you have a higher CO_2 tolerance.
5. If your ***brain-breath connection*** is set to "high" then you have lower amounts of CO_2. This means your body is not familiar with CO_2. Thus, you have a lower CO_2 tolerance. This is what happens in sleep apnea.
6. With a lower CO_2 tolerance, you will feel the urge to breathe much faster when you hold your breath. This is what the relaxed pause measures.

7. Thus, a lower relaxed pause means you have a lower CO_2 tolerance, which means you have been breathing faster and, thus, blocking off your airways.
8. When you increase your relaxed pause, that means you raise your CO_2 tolerance and slow down your nighttime breathing. As a result, you decrease snoring and apnea episodes.

If you noticed, this is still the same concept as the seesaw I described earlier, but with many more steps in between.

As an additional side note, don't worry about CO2 levels being too high. You will not be able to get CO2 levels dangerously high with these exercises. Physiologically, you're just raising your CO2 levels back into a normal range because they're likely a bit too low right now.

Let's Measure Your Relaxed Pause

1. Get Comfortable: Sit down in a comfy chair and relax.
2. Breathe Normally: Breathe in and out through your nose like you usually do for about a minute.
3. Exhale Normally: Take a normal breath in, then breathe out naturally.
4. Hold Your Breath: After you exhale, pinch your nose to hold your breath and start a timer.

5. Feel the Need to Breathe: Hold your breath until you feel the first need to breathe or feel a bit uncomfortable.

6. Stop and Record: Stop the timer and write down how many seconds you held your breath. This is your relaxed pause time.

"What is the first urge to breathe?"

I get this question once a week while working with my clients in our Q&A sessions. Let's start with what the "first urge" is *not*:

1. You should *not* fight or push yourself to hold your breath. That's why I call it a *relaxed* pause.

2. Sometimes people feel a natural pull or tug in their diaphragm, chest, or even throat to breathe within one to five seconds of exhaling. This is just the momentum of your breathing cycle. This is just like the momentum you have when walking that makes it easy to take one step after the other. As a result, this is not the first urge to breathe.

3. Sometimes people may feel a tightness in their throat in the first one to fifteen seconds. This is often the throat muscles having a little twitch that is not problematic. This is not the first urge to breathe.

There are two main ways for someone to get familiar with this first urge to breathe.

1. Get familiar with a warm, slightly uncomfortable feeling in the middle of your chest that radiates as you hold your breath after an exhale. This is quite literally the buildup of carbon dioxide. As soon as you feel this, you have your first urge to breathe.

2. If you can normally inhale and normally exhale for at least five cycles after your relaxed pause, then that means you did not overdo it. If you need a big inhale after measuring your relaxed pause, then you held your breath for too long. So, as your experiment with recording your relaxed pause, you want to correlate how you feel with how you breathe after measuring your relaxed pause.

Here's What Your Relaxed Pause Means

If it makes you feel better, my relaxed pause was between seven to nine seconds when I started measuring. I've been able to get mine to sixty seconds (not necessary for everyone) and it's common for our clients to reach forty-five. Here's a breakdown of the categories and what they mean for you:

Relaxed Pause (seconds)	What It Means
0-10	Severe breathing issues at night
11-20	You'll start to feel improvements in sleep
21-30	This is when you'll notice less snoring and significantly improved sleep
31-40	This is when we typically guide clients in getting off CPAP
41+	This is typically when we see clients start to eliminate sleep apnea fully

Table 5-2: Relaxed pause duration and breathing health

How to Start Improving Your Breathing

You should pick your exercise based on your relaxed pause.

Relaxed Pause (seconds)	Breathing Exercise
<10	10 In 10 Out Breathing
10-15	Box Breathing
>15	Rectangle Breathing

Table 5-3: Relaxed pause duration and associated breathing exercises

Let's go over the breathing routines next:

10 In 10 Out Breathing

Purpose: This exercise promotes relaxation and enhances lung capacity by focusing on deep, controlled breathing. It helps to reduce stress, improve respiratory function, and gradually increase tolerance to carbon dioxide (CO_2) buildup in the body.

1. Find a Comfortable Position:
- Sit or lie down in a comfortable position with your back straight.
- Close your eyes to help focus your attention inward.

2. Inhale Slowly and Deeply:
- Begin by inhaling slowly and deeply through your nose for a count of ten seconds.
- Visualize your lungs filling up with air, expanding your chest and abdomen.

3. Exhale Slowly:
- Exhale slowly through your nose for a count of ten seconds.

4. Continue the Cycle:
- Repeat steps 2 and 3 for five to ten minutes.
- Maintain a smooth and steady rhythm, focusing on the sensation of your breath.

Dylan Petkus

Tips:

- If ten seconds feels too long, start with a count of five and gradually increase as you become more comfortable.
- Place one hand on your abdomen to feel the rise and fall with each breath, ensuring you are breathing deeply.

Box Breathing

Purpose: Also known as four-square breathing, this technique helps to calm the mind, reduce stress, and improve concentration while increasing CO_2 tolerance through controlled breath holds.

1. Find a Quiet Space:
- Sit in a comfortable chair with your feet flat on the ground.
- Close your eyes and relax your shoulders.

2. Inhale Slowly:
- Inhale slowly and deeply through your nose for a count of five seconds.
- Focus on filling your lungs completely.

3. Hold Your Breath:
- Hold your breath for a count of five seconds.

- During this hold, CO_2 levels will rise slightly, helping to build tolerance.

4. Exhale Slowly:

- Exhale slowly through your nose for a count of five seconds.
- Release all the air from your lungs, allowing CO_2 levels to reset.

5. Hold After Exhale:

- Hold your breath for another count of five seconds after the exhale.
- This hold further helps in adapting to increased CO_2 levels.

6. Repeat the Process:

- Repeat steps 2 through 5 for five to ten minutes.
- Focus on the rhythm and steadiness of your breath.

Tips:

- Visualize a box or square, tracing its edges in your mind as you breathe.
- Use this technique before stressful situations to center yourself.

Rectangle Breathing

Purpose: This exercise extends the breath-holding phases, which helps to increase lung capacity and enhance relaxation while significantly improving CO_2 tolerance.

1. Get Comfortable:
- Sit or lie down in a comfortable, quiet place.
- Close your eyes to minimize distractions.

2. Inhale Deeply:
- Inhale slowly and deeply through your nose for a count of five seconds.
- Visualize your lungs filling up completely.

3. Hold Your Breath:
- Hold your breath for a count of ten seconds.
- During this hold, CO_2 levels will rise, helping to build tolerance.

4. Exhale Slowly:
- Exhale slowly through your nose for a count of five seconds.
- Focus on emptying your lungs fully, allowing CO_2 levels to reset.

5. Hold After Exhale:
- Hold your breath for another count of ten seconds after the exhale.
- This extended hold further helps in adapting to increased CO_2 levels.

6. Repeat the Sequence:

- Repeat steps 2 through 5 for five to ten minutes.
- Keep a steady and controlled rhythm throughout.

Tips:

- Visualize a rectangle, with the longer sides representing the breath holds and the shorter sides representing the inhales and exhales.
- Adjust the timing if needed; the goal is to maintain comfort and control.

Implementing the Exercises

1. Decide to do these every time you lie down in bed at night. This maximizes the effectiveness of the routine.
2. Bonus points: you can do another session during the day to help boost your success. Another great time is first thing in the morning to set your breathing for the day.

If You're Using a CPAP

All you need to do differently is do these exercises before you put on your CPAP. Then, when you finish, you put your mask on as usual. Doing these exercises will help make your CPAP work more efficiently. Be patient in your progress and we'll talk about weaning off a CPAP safely in a bit.

The Advantages Of Directly Retraining Your Breathing

These breathing exercises are a huge help in going from a *fragile* approach for sleep apnea with CPAPs, mouth guards, etc. to an approach focused on *building resiliency.* These exercises help build resiliency because of the effect they also have on oxygen which we haven't mentioned yet. As you do these exercises, if you were to wear a pulse oximeter (that thing they put on your finger to measure your blood oxygen levels), you would see slight dips in your oxygen levels. Now, these dips are perfectly fine because they're not as big as the dips you have at night.

In fact, these small oxygen level dips in a controlled environment allow you to build resiliency. I know this may sound counterintuitive because we're told that the dips in oxygen at night hurt our bodies. This is true, but it's an oversimplification. The important detail is that it's the big swings in oxygen levels that go on for hours at night that cause all the damage of sleep apnea. This damage happens in every organ in your body, from your brain to your heart.[21]

When these swings in oxygen happen throughout the entire night, that is too much for your body to handle.

21 Gabryelska A et al. Obstructive Sleep Apnea: From Intermittent Hypoxia to Cardiovascular Complications via Blood Platelets. Front Neurol. 2018 Aug 3;9:635.

But, when you give your body a tiny bit of these low oxygen levels, this helps make your cells more resilient.[22,23] In fact, such low oxygen training has been shown to reverse the high blood pressure in patients with sleep apnea by up to ten blood pressure points on systolic (the top number).[24]

Making your body resilient to low oxygen levels is just like working out. If you lifted weights for eight hours a day, the only thing you would accomplish is breaking down your body. However, if you lift weights strategically, then your body responds positively. That's why if you lower your oxygen levels strategically during the day with these breathing exercises, it will make your body more resilient to the oxygen swings at night.

That's what makes these breathing exercises so effective. Not only do they target the root issue, but they also make you more resilient to the damage of sleep apnea. And, once again, these breathing exercises work with all anatomical issues. Remember, this approach is about working with your anatomy, not against it!

22 Burtscher J et al. Adaptive Responses to Hypoxia and/or Hyperoxia in Humans. Antioxid Redox Signal. 2022 Nov;37(13-15):887-912.

23 Zhang Q et al. Intermittent Hypoxia Conditioning: A Potential Multi-Organ Protective Therapeutic Strategy. Int J Med Sci. 2023 Sep 18;20(12):1551-1561.

24 Panza GS et al. Daily Exposure to Mild Intermittent Hypoxia Reduces Blood Pressure in Male Patients with Obstructive Sleep Apnea and Hypertension. Am J Respir Crit Care Med. 2022 Apr 15;205(8):949-958.

How Do You Know This Is Working?

Here are a few signs you're moving in the right direction:

- You'll feel a sense of calm and slower breathing after you do the exercises.
- If you have trouble falling asleep, this will help you drift off to sleep much faster.
- If you're using a CPAP, it can start to feel easier to use. Or you may see a lower AHI reading on it.
- If you snore, this can help you snore less whether it's something you record or your partner tells you.
- If you wake up a ton in the middle of the night gasping for air, this can decrease these episodes.

Roadblocks Ahead

First, I want to be clear that some, but not all, have overnight results. There are a few reasons you will hit a wall:

- You're doing the exercises wrong. Sorry, but this is one of the most common mistakes our clients make. Make sure you're doing them correctly as outlined above or in the audio tracks below.
- There is something highly individual to you that is making the breathing exercises less effective, such as anatomical variations or certain breathing pattern problems. I know earlier I said these exercises work for all anatomical variations. However,

there are exercises that are best for people with nasal issues, exercises best for those with tongue issues, and so on and so forth. Figuring this out for my clients is a big part of what I do.

- Issues with the other factors can be hurting your breathing so much that the breathing exercises don't have the desired impact. This is similar to the above point. I often need to troubleshoot for clients and help identify which of the other factors is holding them back from progressing their breathing exercises.
- The breathing exercises are not correctly matched with your current level. There is a balance between challenging yourself and pushing too hard. This is another aspect I'm constantly helping clients get comfortable with.
- You need to progress your exercises. One of my biggest goals is to make sure clients are continuing to progress in their breathing exercises. There are all sorts of variations one can add to a single breathing exercise and there are more advanced breathing exercises that require good guidance to ensure safe progression.

As we wrap up this chapter, it's important to acknowledge that your healing journey may require you to step out of your comfort zone. Whether you're engaging in breathing exercises or any other efforts to invest more time, money, and effort into your goals, some discomfort is inevitable. But remember, on the other side of that discomfort lies the restful sleep and energy that you're striving for.

So, take a breather (pun highly intended) and make sure you take advantage of the bonus a couple of pages from here that includes the MP3 downloads for the breathing routines. If you like relaxing music and someone counting for you, then you'll love these audio tracks.

Client Highlight: Mike's Journey to Better Sleep

"The breathing exercises were a game changer. Within a week, I slept six straight hours, something I hadn't experienced in years. My focus and energy levels skyrocketed."

Our client Mike, 58, from Tampa, Florida

Mike, an accountant known for his diligence, struggled with the cumbersome CPAP machine that did little to improve his condition. Despite using it consistently, he woke up unrefreshed, foggy, and fatigued. His work performance suffered, and he felt like he was drowning in an ocean of fatigue, desperate to reclaim his mental sharpness.

One particularly bad night, Mike woke up gasping for breath with his heart pounding. His doctor warned him about the serious health risks if his sleep apnea wasn't properly managed. Desperate for a solution, Mike considered the Inspire implant but was deterred by the thought of painful surgery and complications.

Finding hope in this book, Mike began practicing the breathing exercises. Though initially hesitant, he saw small improvements. Realizing he needed expert guidance, Mike scheduled a free evaluation call and decided to enroll in the program.

With a tailored plan of breathing and airway exercises, Mike slept for six straight hours within a week. His work performance improved, and he felt more focused and energized. However, he started to stall a bit in his progress. So, that's when we continued to update and optimize his protocol. That's how a few months later Mike's sleep apnea had improved so much that he no longer needed his CPAP machine.

As a result, Mike was happy to pack up and return that dreaded machine. Now instead he is sleeping quietly and waking up refreshed just like he used to.

MP3 Downloads So You Can Easily Follow Along With The Breathing Exercises

It is one thing to know how to do an exercise and another to have everything you need to make it happen on a regular basis. That's why I made MP3 audio files. All you have to do is download them, press "play," and follow along.

Use the link below to get a PDF that includes links to the breathing exercises I've mentioned above. Remember, the links to the MP3s are in the PDF!

Click here to get them:

TheSleepApneaSolution.com/breathing

Or use your phone's camera to focus on the QR code below, and touch the link that pops up on your phone to help you access the breathing exercises:

Top Breathing Tips

1. Nasal Breathing

Why: Nasal breathing releases nitric oxide, which helps open the airways, improving airflow and reducing the risk of sleep apnea episodes. *If you have snoring, then this is critically important!*

How: Practice keeping your mouth closed and breathing through your nose throughout the day and night. If you struggle with nasal congestion, consider using a saline spray or a nasal strip to keep your nasal passages clear.

2. Diaphragm Breathing

Why: Diaphragm (or belly) breathing promotes deeper breaths and enhances lung capacity, which can improve oxygen levels during sleep.

How: Lie on your back with one hand on your chest and the other on your abdomen. Inhale deeply through your nose, ensuring your abdomen rises more than your chest. Exhale slowly through your mouth. Practice this for a few minutes each day, particularly before bedtime.

3. Posture

Why: Good posture helps maintain open airways, reducing the likelihood of airway obstruction during sleep.

How: During the day, practice sitting and standing with a straight back and relaxed shoulders. While sleeping, try to avoid positions that could cause your tongue and soft tissues to block your airway. Sleeping on your side can be particularly beneficial for reducing sleep apnea symptoms.

4. Reassess Your Relaxed Pause Every Day

Why: This helps give you a good idea of your progress.

How: Ideally, do this at the same time every morning. You can get away with just one measurement. But I recommend taking three measurements and then averaging them.

CPAP Freedom Roadmap:

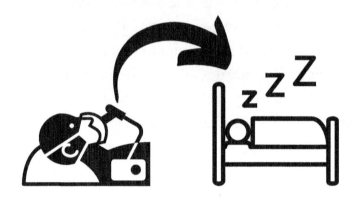

Now that you have a way to improve your nighttime breathing, I want to show you how I guide my clients in breaking free from their CPAP. I've noticed people have two main frustrations with CPAP:

1. They use their CPAP consistently but still feel awful.
2. They feel fine but hate their CPAP.

It's tricky because we all want to feel better, but the idea of leaving our CPAP behind can be scary. You might have heard the warning, *"You have to use your CPAP, or you're going to die."*

Now, I'm **not** saying CPAPs don't help some people. Some individuals are so happy with their CPAPs that they even name them! And that is fine.

However, if you're here, it's likely because a CPAP isn't working for you. Or, you hate having to use one.

That's why I want to show you that breaking free from your CPAP can be relatively easy and, more importantly, safe! Click the link below to get your exclusive access to the CPAP Freedom Roadmap video and PDF. Take the first step toward better sleep and reclaiming your freedom today!

TheSleepApneaSolution.com/freedom

Here's your QR code to scan if you'd like:

Help Others With Sleep Apnea And Get A Free Gift:

As you're a little more than halfway through the book, I'm hoping you can help me and everyone with sleep apnea. You see, there are about 30,000,000 people with sleep apnea in the United States alone.

It's our mission to make this book as helpful and powerful as possible. We'd really appreciate your feedback on what's been helpful for you so far. All you need to do is complete a super short survey.

And, once you complete it, I'll give you a free gift as a "thank you."

So, kindly click the link below or type it into your browser:

TheSleepApneaSolution.com/thanks

And, if you prefer to use a QR code, please scan below to access the survey and receive your gift.

Chapter 6
Nutrition

As we continue our journey to address sleep apnea, I want to re-emphasize how directly working on your breathing patterns with exercises is only thirty to forty percent of the battle. The other four factors we're about to dive into next make up the rest of your full recovery.

The first factor we're going to tackle is nutrition specific to sleep apnea. Generally good nutrition is not what we're talking about here. I've had many clients that come to me who eat like a certified health nut and swear that their diet is amazing! However, again, any diet for general good health may have some benefit for sleep apnea, but it will not specifically target your sleep apnea needs. To fully address sleep apnea through nutrition, it's essential to understand the underlying issues that sleep apnea causes within the body.

What happens at a high level is that sleep apnea events cause inflammation. This inflammation depletes you of micronutrients (vitamins and minerals). The decrease in micronutrients forces you to be a sugar burner. All of which makes your breathing at night even worse and further contributes to a negative cycle of even more sleep apnea events, as shown below:

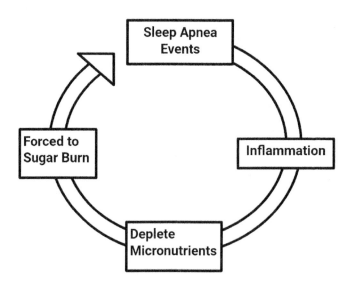

Figure 6-14: Cycle of sleep apnea and impaired nutrition

So, all we need to do is break this cycle to reduce the negative downward spiral. Let's talk about each component a bit more in-depth below.

Sleep Apnea Inflammation

When your body is attacked by constant oxygen level swings resulting from poor breathing at night, this causes widespread inflammation. That's why, when doctors and researchers look at inflammatory markers in the blood, they are significantly higher in patients with sleep apnea.[25] Think of inflammation like a fire in your cells. In fact, a house fire is a pretty good analogy for how your entire body is right now. When things are ablaze, they don't work quite as well. Brain inflamed? You can barely think straight. Heart inflamed? Blood pressure goes up. Muscles inflamed? You feel heavy and sluggish.

When your body is inflamed, it enters into an emergency state of metabolism. This then depletes micronutrients. Let's talk about that next.

Sleep Apnea Inflammation Depletes Certain Micronutrients

Micronutrients are small substances like vitamins and minerals that are essential for your body's function. Research shows widespread inflammation can deplete many key nutrients.[26,27] These depleted nutrients can include:

25 Suša R et al. Does the Severity of Obstructive Sleep Apnea Have an Independent Impact on Systemic Inflammation? Medicina (Kaunas). 2021 Mar 22;57(3):292.

26 Peuhkuri K, Sihvola N, Korpela R. Diet promotes sleep duration and quality. Nutr Res. 2012 May;32(5):309-19.

27 Breuillard C et al. Chronic intermittent hypoxia due to obstructive sleep apnea slightly alters nutritional status: a pre-clinical study. Front Nutr. 2023 Oct 30;10:1250529.

- **Magnesium:** Essential for muscle and nerve function. A deficiency can lead to increased stress and poor sleep quality.
- **B Vitamins** (especially B6, B12, and folic acid): Crucial for energy production, red blood cell formation, and neurological function. Deficiencies can result in fatigue and cognitive impairments.
- **Zinc:** Important for immune function and protein synthesis. Low levels can impair immune response and wound healing.
- **Iron:** Necessary for production of hemoglobin and overall energy levels. Deficiency can cause anemia and chronic fatigue.
- **Vitamin C and E:** These antioxidants help combat oxidative stress. Inflammation can reduce their levels, leading to increased oxidative damage.

One-thing-itis Alert

Now, don't go out and get supplements to cover all of these. That puts you back into one-thing-itis thinking! These are some of the most common deficiencies that happen in someone with sleep apnea. However, as I've noticed in our clients, everyone has their own set of deficiencies that we can pick up in our initial assessment process. Lastly, when improving micronutrient status, I always prefer to do that by including certain foods. Only when I feel we're falling short with food alone will I recommend specific supplements for individual cases.

These deficiencies lead to you becoming a sugar burner. Let's talk about that next.

Sleep Apnea Forces You to Be A Sugar Burner

Ideally, you will burn sugar (carbohydrate), protein, and fat as fuel sources in your body. However, when you have inflammation and micronutrient issues, they hurt your metabolism. What happens is that your cells become worse at fat burning. That's why the research has shown that people with sleep apnea burn half as much fat as people without sleep apnea.[28]

When your body can't burn fat, it will default to burning sugar. This means your body relies more heavily on glucose for energy, leading to increased carbohydrate cravings. When your body defaults to burning sugar, you may experience frequent energy crashes and a constant need to replenish your sugar levels. This can create a vicious cycle of craving and consuming more

---

28 Schmidt F et al. Severe Obstructive Sleep Apnea Disrupts Vigilance-State-Dependent Metabolism. Int J Mol Sci. 2022 Nov 14;23(22):14052.

carbohydrates, which can lead to further metabolic imbalances and weight gain.

Moreover, relying on sugar as a primary energy source can result in unstable blood sugar levels. These fluctuations can lead to feelings of fatigue, irritability, and difficulty concentrating, further disrupting your sleep patterns and overall health. If you find yourself frequently craving carbohydrates, especially sugary snacks or high-carb foods, it's a clear sign that your body is stuck in sugar-burning mode due to the metabolic disruptions caused by sleep apnea.

These Metabolic Problems Make Breathing at Night Even Worse

The metabolic issues caused by sleep apnea and the shift toward sugar-burning then worsens breathing at night.[29] When your body relies heavily on sugar for energy, it results in frequent spikes and crashes in blood sugar levels. These fluctuations can lead to periods of low blood sugar during the night, which can disrupt your sleep and cause your body to release stress hormones like cortisol and adrenaline. These hormones can stimulate your nervous system, **which makes your breathing faster and causes more snoring and apnea episodes.**

29 Framnes SN et al. The Bidirectional Relationship Between Obstructive Sleep Apnea and Metabolic Disease. Front Endocrinol (Lausanne). 2018 Aug 6;9:440.

Additionally, the inflammation associated with sleep apnea can further impair your respiratory system. Inflammation in the upper airway tissues can lead to swelling and increased airway resistance, making it more difficult to breathe effectively during sleep. This increased airway resistance can worsen the severity of obstructive sleep apnea, leading to more frequent interruptions in breathing and further disrupting your sleep quality.

Moreover, the weight gain associated with a high-sugar diet can contribute to the severity of sleep apnea. Excess weight, particularly around the neck and abdomen, can increase the pressure on your airway and diaphragm, making it harder for you to breathe comfortably at night.

So, it is super clear we have some unique metabolic issues we need to unravel so that you will breathe slower at night and keep your airways open.

How Can We Begin to Fix These Issues?

Optimizing your protein intake and reducing inflammatory food consumption are the two best ways to start reversing these metabolic issues and improve breathing at night.

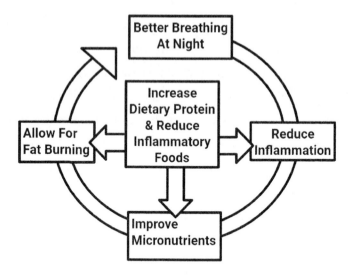

Figure 6-15: Benefits of increased dietary protein and reduced inflammation

Reducing inflammatory foods (as we'll discuss below) and increasing dietary protein intake are crucial steps in addressing the metabolic issues caused by sleep apnea. These dietary changes can help reverse inflammation, correct micronutrient deficiencies, and shift your body from being a forced sugar burner toward a more balanced state of metabolism.

1. Reducing Inflammation

Inflammation is a key factor that exacerbates sleep apnea and its related metabolic issues. By reducing inflammation, you can improve your body's ability to absorb and utilize essential nutrients more effectively.

When inflammation is reduced, the upper airway tissues become less swollen, decreasing airway resistance and making breathing easier during sleep. Additionally, lower inflammation levels can help regulate cortisol production, leading to more stable blood sugar levels and, thus, stable breathing at night.

2. Increasing Dietary Protein

Increasing your intake of protein-rich foods addresses several critical metabolic issues associated with sleep apnea. High-quality protein sources provide many of the essential amino acids and micronutrients that are depleted in sleep apnea.

Protein helps stabilize blood sugar levels by slowing down the digestion and absorption of carbohydrates, preventing the rapid rise and fall of blood sugar that can lead to cravings and energy crashes. This stabilization reduces the reliance on sugar as a primary energy source, helping to shift your body toward burning fat more efficiently.

Moreover, protein is essential for muscle repair and maintenance. Adequate protein intake ensures that your body has the necessary building blocks to repair tissue and maintain muscle mass, which is particularly important for individuals with sleep apnea who experience increased metabolic demands and muscle breakdown due to disrupted sleep.

How This Helps Breathing at Night

By reducing inflammation and increasing dietary protein, you address the root causes of the metabolic imbalances that worsen sleep apnea. Here's how these changes ultimately improve your breathing at night:

- **Reduced Airway Resistance:** Lower inflammation levels decrease swelling in the upper airway tissues, reducing airway resistance and making it easier to breathe during sleep.
- **Stable Blood Sugar Levels:** Balanced blood sugar levels prevent nighttime hypoglycemic episodes, reducing the release of stress hormones that can disrupt sleep and cause more frequent apnea episodes.
- **Enhanced Fat Burning:** Shifting your body from being a forced sugar burner to efficiently burning fat reduces metabolic stress and supports sustained energy levels throughout the night.

By incorporating more protein-rich foods and reducing inflammatory foods in your diet, you can break the cycle of metabolic dysfunction, support your body's natural healing processes, and achieve better sleep quality. Let's dice into exactly how you can do that.

Foods to Exclude for Reducing Airway Inflammation

Dairy Products
Dairy products such as milk and yogurt are common culprits when it comes to airway inflammation. For many people, dairy can increase mucus production, leading to congestion and inflammation in the airways. This can make breathing more difficult, especially at night.

How to Manage:
- Replace Cow's Milk: Try almond milk or oat milk as alternatives.
- Choose Non-Dairy Yogurts: Look for yogurt made from coconut milk or almond milk.

What about cheese?
Although cheese is indeed dairy, I don't find it to cause much inflammation in the airways of patients. I believe this is due to the fact it has less contact than a liquid (milk or yogurt) would have. So, you can keep your cheese!

Coffee and Caffeine
While a morning cup of coffee can feel like a necessity, caffeine can have inflammatory effects on the airways. Caffeine is a stimulant that can increase heart rate and

disrupt sleep patterns, potentially worsening sleep apnea symptoms.

How to Manage:
- *Limit Intake:* If you can't give up coffee entirely, try to limit your intake to one cup a day, preferably in the morning.
- *Choose Alternatives:* Consider drinking herbal teas or decaffeinated coffee instead.
- *Hydrate:* Ensure you're drinking plenty of water throughout the day to stay hydrated and support overall health. A good rule of thumb is half your body weight (in pounds) in ounces. For example, a 180-pound man should strive to drink ninety ounces of water per day.

Cut Out Processed Foods
Processed foods often contain additives, preservatives, and unhealthy fats that can contribute to inflammation.

How to Manage:
- *Read Labels:* Avoid foods with long ingredient lists, especially those with additives and preservatives.
- *Cook at Home:* Preparing meals at home allows you to control the ingredients and avoid processed foods.

Alcohol and Sleep Apnea
Alcohol can significantly impact sleep apnea by both causing inflammation in the airways and overly relaxing the muscles, leading to increased airway collapse. Here's

how alcohol affects sleep apnea and how you can manage its intake to improve your condition.

How Alcohol Affects Sleep Apnea

Inflammation: Alcohol can cause inflammation throughout the body, including in the airways. This inflammation can lead to swelling and congestion, making it harder to breathe properly and exacerbating sleep apnea symptoms.

Muscle Relaxation: While you might think a nightcap can help you relax, alcohol actually relaxes the muscles in your throat and upper airway too much. This excessive relaxation can cause the airways to collapse more easily during sleep, leading to more frequent apneas.

Disrupted Sleep Patterns: Alcohol can disrupt your sleep architecture, reducing the quality of your sleep. It can prevent you from reaching the deeper stages of sleep, which are essential for restorative rest and recovery. This leads to poorer sleep quality and worsens the effects of sleep apnea.

Dehydration: Alcohol can dehydrate the body, and dehydration can thicken the mucus in your airways, further obstructing breathing and exacerbating sleep apnea.

What the Research Says About Alcohol:

Studies have shown that alcohol consumption before bedtime increases the severity and frequency of obstructive sleep apnea events. Alcohol-induced relaxation of the upper airway muscles is a significant factor in this increased severity. Additionally, research indicates that even moderate alcohol consumption can lead to inflammation and disrupted sleep patterns, worsening sleep apnea symptoms.[30]

How to Manage Alcohol Intake

- **Set Boundaries**: If you consume alcohol, try to limit it to one drink per day.

- **Avoid Late-Night Drinks**: Avoid drinking alcohol within three to four hours of bedtime to minimize its impact on your sleep and airway muscles.

- **Opt for Non-Alcoholic Beverages**: Consider drinking non-alcoholic beverages such as sparkling water, herbal teas, or non-alcoholic beers and wines.

- **Mocktails**: Enjoy non-alcoholic cocktails that provide the same social experience without the negative effects on your sleep.

Research Detour

A study conducted at Harvard Medical School examined 8,856 people with sleep apnea over ten years. They found that low-inflammatory diets led to a twenty-four percent reduction in sleep

---

30 Ko J et al. Association between alcohol use disorder and risk of obstructive sleep apnea. J Sleep Res. 2024 Aug;33(4):e14128.

apnea severity. Conversely, the severity of sleep apnea increased by ninety-four percent with a more pro-inflammatory diet.[31] By increasing protein intake and reducing inflammatory foods, you can lower inflammation and significantly improve sleep apnea symptoms.

Proteins to Include for Better Breathing At Night

To improve your breathing at night and support overall health, incorporate the following protein-rich foods into your diet:

- Lean Meats: Chicken, turkey, and lean cuts of beef and pork are excellent sources of high-quality protein.
- Fish: Salmon, mackerel, and sardines are not only rich in protein but also contain omega-3 fatty acids, which help reduce inflammation.
- Eggs: A versatile and nutrient-dense option that provides essential amino acids and vitamins.
- Protein powders: Whey, casein, etc. can all be easy additions to increase dietary protein.

---

31 Liu Y et al. Overall diet quality and proinflammatory diet in relation to risk of obstructive sleep apnea in 3 prospective US cohorts. Am J Clin Nutr. 2022 Dec 19;116(6):1738-1747.

How Do You Know This Is Working?

Again, the below won't happen after eating one chicken breast, but you can begin to feel a bit of the following as you start:

- Improved energy levels throughout the day.
- Reduced cravings for sugary snacks and high-carb foods.
- More stable blood sugar levels, leading to fewer energy crashes.
- Better muscle maintenance and less fatigue.
- Enhanced sleep quality with fewer disruptions.
- Reduced frequency of nighttime awakenings and apnea episodes.
- Overall feeling of better health and well-being.

Roadblocks Ahead

As with anything, you may run into some walls in your journey:

- **Individual Nutrient Needs:** Some individuals have more specific nutrient needs that we figure out with our clients. This could mean tailoring protein sources or supplementing certain vitamins and minerals.
- **Digestive Issues:** Incorporating more protein can sometimes cause digestive discomfort if not done gradually.

- **Balancing Macronutrients:** Finding the right balance of proteins, fats, and carbohydrates can be challenging.
- **Sustaining Changes:** Maintaining dietary changes can be difficult without ongoing support. This is why our team devotes time to coaching our clients; just because you know better doesn't mean you do better.

Wrapping Up This Chapter

Addressing sleep apnea through nutrition is a powerful step toward better health and improved sleep quality. By reducing inflammation and increasing your intake of protein-rich foods, you can correct metabolic imbalances, enhance your body's nutrient absorption, and support more effective breathing at night. Remember, the journey to better sleep starts with actionable dietary changes that you can implement today. Don't forget to download the protein checklist at the end of this chapter for easy tips and meal ideas to help you get started. Here's to a healthier, more restful night's sleep!

Client Highlight: Kevin's Journey to Better Sleep

"One thing I did differently was change my food, which really changed things for the better. My sleep apnea got a lot better. I started sleeping a lot better. And my energy level, whoa, my energy level went through the roof with the right kind of foods."

Our client Kevin, 62, from Chicago, Illinois

Kevin dreaded his nightly routine with his wife Julie, as the noise of his CPAP machine made sleeping together impossible. Julie often retreated to the guest room, leaving Kevin feeling isolated and less like a husband. Despite his efforts, Kevin would wake up unrefreshed, and Julie's disappointment was palpable each morning when she saw he had removed the CPAP during the night.

One morning, Kevin found Julie quietly crying at the kitchen table, overwhelmed by his suffering. This moment was a wake-up call for Kevin. Determined to change, he promised Julie they would figure it out together. However, Kevin's attempts with various mouthguards and gadgets failed, leaving him disheartened.

Kevin stumbled upon our program and, despite his doubts, decided to give it a try. He initially saw small improvements but struggled without a cohesive plan. Julie encouraged him to seek personalized support, and Kevin finally booked an evaluation call with us. During the call, he felt understood and hopeful for the first time in years.

With a personalized nutrition plan, Kevin cut out inflammatory foods and started seeing subtle improvements, like less brain fog and more energy for date nights. However, Kevin hit a stumbling block when he struggled with persistent sugar cravings that derailed his progress. Through our guidance, we tailored his diet further and introduced specific protein-rich foods to stabilize his blood sugar levels. This made all the difference and allowed him to eventually ditch his CPAP.

Without the CPAP between them, Kevin and Julie finally slept together peacefully. As restful sleep became routine, Kevin's confidence and vitality returned, rekindling their relationship and allowing them to dream of the future together.

Exclusive Book Bonus:
Protein Made Easy

As a special bonus, you're getting an exclusive guide that makes implementing this chapter easy. This bonus material breaks down the essentials of incorporating protein into your diet without the need for complicated recipes or hard-to-find ingredients.

Inside this guide, you'll discover:

1. Simple meal ideas that require minimal preparation and cooking time.
2. Protein-rich snack suggestions to keep you satisfied between meals.
3. Tips for meeting your protein needs while eating out or on-the-go.

Click below to get your exclusive book bonus:

TheSleepApneaSolution.com/protein

And, of course, you can scan the QR code here:

Chapter 7
Circadian Rhythm

Your circadian rhythm is how your body properly times all the different biological processes. Think of it as your body's internal clock that tells you when to wake up, when to eat, and when to go to sleep. Just like how a real clock tells you what time of day it is, your circadian rhythm helps your body know what time it is so it can do things at the right times. For example, it helps you feel sleepy at night and awake during the day. It also makes sure your body releases certain hormones, like cortisol (which makes you alert in the morning) and melatonin (which helps you sleep at night) at the right times.

When your circadian rhythm is off, your body's internal clock gets confused. This can make you feel tired during the day and wide awake at night, similar to the feeling of jet lag. You might have trouble falling asleep or waking up at the right times. It can also disrupt other things, like making you feel hungry at odd times or affecting your mood, making you feel irritable or down. Just like how you might struggle to adjust if your work schedule suddenly changes, your body has a hard time functioning properly when its internal clock is out of sync.

Sleep Apnea And Your Circadian Rhythm

Sleep apnea completely destroys your body's circadian rhythm which then makes sleep apnea even worse. In fact, this is such a big part of the problem some research experts are suggesting that sleep apnea should be considered a circadian rhythm disorder.[32]

When your circadian rhythm is off, it makes your sleep quality even worse. That is, when you aren't suffocating yourself at night, the sleep you do get is low quality. That's why people with sleep apnea may find it harder to fall asleep, stay asleep, or get restful sleep. This is also why people who use a CPAP, but still have a poor circadian rhythm, continue to have unrefreshing sleep.

Not only will a bad circadian rhythm lead to poor sleep quality, but it will also contribute to worse breathing at night as well. Research shows that disrupted circadian rhythms can make sleep apnea worse by affecting the

---

32 Šmon J et al. Is obstructive sleep apnea a circadian rhythm disorder? J Sleep Res. 2023 Aug;32(4):e13875.

body's natural control over breathing patterns during sleep.[33] Circadian misalignment has been linked to increased airway resistance and reduced respiratory muscle efficiency, making it harder to maintain stable breathing during sleep.[31]

Over time, the cycle perpetuates itself. A disrupted circadian rhythm leads to bad nights of sleep, which lead to a worse circadian rhythm. It is a dreadful cycle as shown below:

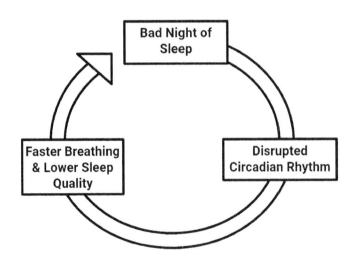

Figure 7-16: Cycle showing negative effects of disrupted circadian rhythm

33 Soreca I. The role of circadian rhythms in Obstructive Sleep Apnea symptoms and novel targets for treatment. Chronobiol Int. 2021 Sep;38(9):1274-1282.

How to Break This Cycle

To break this cycle, you must begin the process of resetting your circadian rhythm, just like you would reset your clock. Once you have a stronger rhythm, you will improve both breathing and sleep quality at night. As a result, you get better sleep, which continues to strengthen your circadian rhythm as shown below:

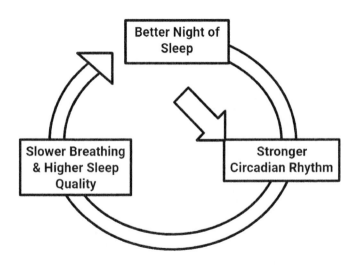

Figure 7-17: Cycle showing positive effects of stronger circadian rhythm

To reset your circadian rhythm, you need to properly time things that give your body signals. These signals help your internal clock understand what time of day it is and what it should be doing. Then, as a result, you have another way to improve your breathing and sleep at night. So, let's discuss the two most important ways to start re-aligning your circadian rhythm.

Step 1: Get Morning Light

Getting morning light is like setting your body's internal alarm clock. Think of your circadian rhythm as a daily schedule that your body follows. When you expose yourself to natural sunlight in the morning, it's like hitting the start button on that schedule. The light signals to your brain that it's time to wake up and be alert.

Morning light helps to set your internal clock by regulating the production of melatonin, the hormone that makes you feel sleepy. During the day, light exposure reduces melatonin levels, helping you stay awake and alert. As the day progresses and light decreases, melatonin levels rise, preparing your body for sleep. This natural rise and fall in melatonin level is crucial for good sleep quality.

By getting sunlight in the morning, you effectively set your internal clock for the day ahead. This not only helps you feel more awake and energetic during the day but also prepares your body for a restful night's sleep. Consistent morning light exposure keeps your circadian rhythm in sync, which in turn improves your breathing at night. When your body knows it's time to sleep, your breathing can become more regular and less disrupted by apnea episodes, leading to better overall sleep quality.

So, think of morning light as the cue that kickstarts your day and sets you up for a good night's sleep. It's a simple yet powerful way to help your body maintain a healthy rhythm and improve your nighttime breathing. In fact, that's why researchers at the University of Pittsburgh found that bright morning light significantly improved sleep quality.[34]

How to Get Morning Light

1. *Go Outside Early:* Spend at least ten to fifteen minutes outside within an hour of waking up. This exposure helps signal to your body that it's time to wake up and start the day.

2. *Open Your Curtains:* If going outside isn't an option, open your curtains wide to let in as much natural light as possible.

That's the basics of step 1. At the end of this chapter, there will be a bonus that goes over many different scenarios on how to make this easy, actionable, and more effective. Now, let's talk about the next step.

---

34 Soreca I, Arnold N, Dombrovski AY. Bright light therapy for CPAP-resistant OSA symptoms. J Clin Sleep Med. 2024 Feb 1;20(2):211-219.

Step 2: Less Light at Night

Just as getting morning light helps set your internal clock for the day, reducing light exposure at night helps prepare your body for sleep. Think of your circadian rhythm as a dimmer switch for your body's activities. In the evening, you need to gradually dim the lights to signal to your brain that it's time to wind down.

One of the most important aspects to improve is the production of melatonin at night—especially for those with sleep apnea. Melatonin is your "sleep hormone." When you have less melatonin, you will have worse sleep quality. Research has shown that people with sleep apnea have fifty percent lower melatonin levels compared to those without it.[35] Thus, people with sleep apnea need to make sure they boost their melatonin levels as much as possible to have higher quality sleep.

Why Not Just Take Melatonin in a Pill?

While it might seem easier to take melatonin supplements, doing so can lead to unnaturally high blood concentrations, making your airway muscles more likely to collapse and potentially causing dependency

---

35 Hernández C et al. Nocturnal melatonin plasma levels in patients with OSAS: the effect of CPAP. Eur Respir J. 2007 Sep;30(3):496-500.

on the supplement. That's why it is important to have lifestyle practices in place to boost your body's own natural ability to make melatonin.

Additionally, when you set your rhythm for the night, this then further helps make sure you have a smooth breathing pattern to reduce apnea episodes at night. So, let's talk about how to set your rhythm for better sleep.

How to Set Your Rhythm For The Night

One of the best ways to boost melatonin naturally is by reducing light exposure at night. In fact, a systematic review found that lowering light exposure at night can improve melatonin levels by twenty-five to fifty percent.[36] Here's how you can easily do this:

1. *Wear Sunglasses at Night:* Wearing sunglasses for two to three hours before bedtime can significantly reduce light exposure. Most people already have sunglasses, making this an easy and effective method.

2. *Dim the Lights:* Use dimmer switches or low-wattage bulbs in the evening to create a calming environment.

3. *Avoid Screens*: Reduce screen time from TVs, phones, and computers at least an hour before bed.

---

36 Tähkämö, L. et al. Systematic review of light exposure impact on human circadian rhythm. Chronobiology International, 2019 36(2), 151–170.

Dylan Petkus

As a quick sidenote, I encourage you to get over the weirdness of wearing sunglasses at night. If we can accept wearing CPAP machines, we can certainly wear sunglasses in the evening. Remember, you'll need to do things few people do to get results few people get.

How Do You Know This Is Working?

From the above action steps, what you can expect is an initial bump followed by subtle shifts, such as:

- You wake up feeling more refreshed and alert in the morning, indicating a well-aligned circadian rhythm.
- Your energy levels remain stable throughout the day without the need for frequent naps or caffeine.
- You find it easier to fall asleep quickly at night and stay asleep until morning.
- Your snoring and apnea episodes decrease in frequency and severity, resulting in fewer nighttime awakenings.

Roadblocks Ahead

Just like anything that seems simple at first, there are many complexities that arise along the way. Here are a few to consider when working to improve your circadian rhythm:

- **Individual Lifestyle Factors:** Many people have unique lifestyle factors, such as irregular work schedules or high stress levels, that can disrupt their circadian rhythm. This is why we help our clients personalize their strategies to address these challenges.
- **Personalized Meal Timing:** Optimizing meal timing to support your circadian rhythm is highly individual.
- **Inconsistent Light Exposure:** It can be difficult to consistently get the right amount of morning light and reduce evening light due to varying daily schedules and commitments. However, with some guidance based on personal needs, we help our clients find workarounds.
- **Underlying Health Issues:** Some individuals may have underlying health conditions that interfere with their circadian rhythm.
- **Habit Formation:** Building new habits around light exposure and sleep routines can be challenging without support.

Wrapping Up This Chapter

In this chapter, we've discussed the importance of your circadian rhythm and how it impacts your sleep quality and breathing. We've explored how increasing morning light exposure and light reduction at night can help reset your internal clock, leading to better overall health. Understanding and optimizing your circadian rhythm is a crucial step in managing sleep apnea and improving your quality of life. In the next chapter, we will dive into the nervous system and its role in sleep apnea. But don't forget your circadian bonus below!

Exclusive Book Bonus: Circadian Rhythm Action Guide

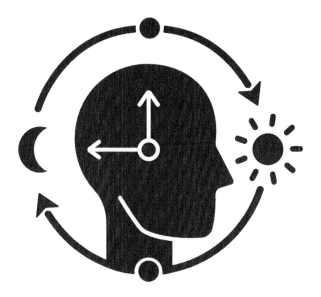

If you want a simple, to-the-point checklist to optimize your circadian rhythm, then use the link below:

TheSleepApneaSolution.com/routines

Or, scan the QR code below for the circadian routine checklist:

Client Highlight: Christina's Journey to Better Sleep

"I didn't realize just how important circadian rhythms were until I began treating them as important, but as soon as I did I almost ceased to snore, and I started to wake up in the morning feeling that I'd had a good night's sleep. I can't believe how much better I sleep."

Our client Christina, 51 from Austin, Texas

Christina dragged herself through each day, hiding her exhaustion with coffee and makeup. Her sleep apnea left her too tired to enjoy playing with her kids and made her irritable and short-tempered. Despite her doctors pushing her to try a CPAP machine, Christina felt overwhelmed and anxious about the idea.

One morning, after a particularly rough night, Christina snapped at her children over a small spill. Seeing the hurt in their eyes and her husband's concern, she knew she needed to make a change.

After discovering our program, Christina scheduled a free evaluation call. During the call, she shared her struggles, and I assured her that with targeted lifestyle changes and airway exercises, she could reverse her sleep apnea. Motivated by the vision of a healthier life, Christina committed to the program.

One of the most significant changes Christina made was optimizing her circadian rhythm. By adjusting the timing of her activities, she aligned her body's natural processes. However, Christina initially struggled with her irregular work schedule, which often kept her up late into the night and left her feeling exhausted during the day. We worked with her to create a personalized plan that included gradually adjusting her sleep and wake times and incorporating morning light exposure. This alignment with her body's natural processes not only gave her more energy and better sleep but also reduced her snoring and apnea episodes. This simple yet powerful adjustment gave her more energy and better sleep.

Within weeks, Christina's exhaustion lifted, and she no longer needed to worry about CPAP therapy. She had the mental clarity and stamina to play with her kids, support her husband, and enjoy her hobbies. By investing in her health, Christina transformed not only her life but also the lives of her family.

Public Service Announcement: Go To Bed at a Reasonable Hour

In going over sleep tracking data for a few clients I noticed a really interesting trend.

I found that the later someone goes to bed, the worse their oxygen saturation levels are at night.

For example, we have one client who, whenever he went to bed at around midnight, would have twice the amount of apnea events.

Even more interesting was that even if he got the same amount of sleep, sleeping later still had a negative effect on his breathing at night.

The reason for this is that when you go to bed later, this will increase the amount of time you spend in REM sleep.

However, when you have too much REM in comparison to the other stages of sleep, this actually makes your breathing worse at night.

Interesting, huh?

No change in anatomy, body position, or anything else.

Just a simple shift in his body's timing (known as his circadian rhythm).

This illustrates 1) why it's important to go to bed earlier and 2) the power of lifestyle changes for sleep apnea.

If you're a night owl, here are some steps to help you get to bed around 9 to 10 p.m.:

Gradual Shift: Start by going to bed fifteen minutes earlier each night. This gradual shift will make the transition easier.

Set a Routine: Establish a calming bedtime routine to signal to your body that it's time to wind down. This could include reading a book, taking a warm bath, or practicing relaxation exercises.

Limit Screen Time: Avoid screens (phones, computers, TVs) at least an hour before bed. The blue light emitted by screens can interfere with your body's production of melatonin, the hormone that regulates sleep.

Create a Sleep-Friendly Environment: Make sure your bedroom is dark, quiet, and cool. Consider using blackout curtains, earplugs, or a white noise machine to create an ideal sleep environment.

Avoid Stimulants: Limit caffeine and nicotine intake in the afternoon and evening. These can keep you awake and disrupt your sleep cycle.

Stay Consistent: Try to wake up and go to bed at the same time every day, even on weekends. Consistency helps regulate your body's internal clock.

Relaxation Techniques: Practice relaxation techniques such as deep breathing, meditation, or progressive muscle relaxation to help calm your mind and body before bed.

Making these changes can significantly improve your sleep quality and reduce the severity of sleep apnea. Remember, small adjustments can lead to big improvements in your health and well-being!

Chapter 8
Nervous System

Sleep apnea disrupts more than just your sleep; it wreaks havoc on your nervous system. Think of your nervous system as the body's control center, managing everything from breathing and heart rate to how you feel and move. Every time you stop breathing during sleep, oxygen levels drop, and this triggers the nervous system to sound the alarm. Your heart races and your blood pressure spikes as your body fights to restore normal breathing. Over time, these repeated episodes can damage the nerves that control your breathing and heart function.[37]

This damage keeps your nervous system in a constant state of overdrive, preventing the deep, restful sleep your body needs. As a result, you may feel tired, cranky, and unfocused during the day. An overactive nervous system

---

37 Venkataraman S et al. Sleep Apnea, Hypertension and the Sympathetic Nervous System in the Adult Population. J Clin Med. 2020 Feb 21;9(2):591.

also worsens nighttime breathing, as damaged nerves fail to control your airway muscles properly, leading to more frequent and severe pauses in breathing. Sleep apnea further harms your nervous system, creating a vicious cycle as shown below:

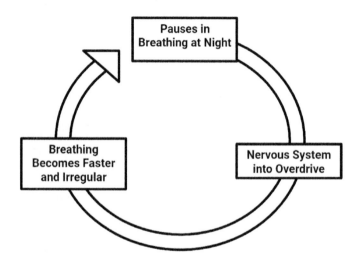

Figure 8-18: Cycle showing negative effects of sleep apnea on the nervous system

Calming your nervous system is key to breaking this cycle. By reducing the stress on your nervous system, you can improve your sleep quality.

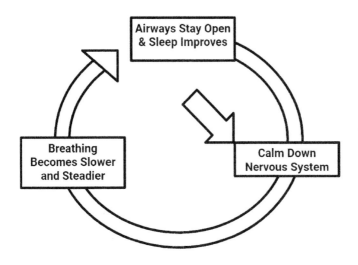

Figure 8-19: Cycle showing positive effects of sleep apnea reduction on the nervous system

Calming down the nervous system is as simple as using relaxation techniques like deep, slow breathing. Gratitude and guided imagery have also been proven to activate the parasympathetic nervous system, promoting relaxation and reducing stress. One study showed that participants who engaged in these mind-body routines reduced their Apnea-Hypopnea Index (AHI), a measure of sleep apnea severity, by half.[38]

---

38 Yilmaz Gokmen G et al. The Effect of T'ai Chi and Qigong Training on Patients with Obstructive Sleep Apnea: A Randomized Controlled Study. J Altern Complement Med. 2019 Mar;25(3):317-325

That's why I want to share the fastest way for anyone (no meditation experience required) to quickly calm your nervous system.

Woo-woo Warning

The following may feel a bit "woo-woo" and that's okay. The practice I'm sharing below is just a highly refined way to accomplish many of the outcomes of relaxing your nervous system. There are a thousand different ways to do this, from prayer to simply journaling. In working with our clients, we find multiple ways that work for them to calm their nervous system.

So, even if you're skeptical or feel this is a bunch of hogwash, I invite you to try out the exercise and get the MP3 at the end of this chapter. Just suspend judgment the first few times and I think you'll be pleasantly surprised with the results.

How to Start Resetting Your Nervous System

I'm going to walk you through step by step for this exercise. At the end of this chapter, there is a bonus download link so you can follow along with my instructions. Here are the steps:

Step 1: Pick Your Gratitude Reset Time

Choose a time in the late morning or early afternoon when your nervous system and you are likely to hit a wall.

Step 2: Download the Gratitude Reset Audio (There is a link at the end of this chapter).

Step 3: Press Play and follow the instructions.

Note: The following steps are provided in an audio-track format to make them easy to follow.

1. Reset Your Breathing Phase

- Find a comfortable position, either sitting or lying down.
- Take a slow, deep breath through your nose, hold for a moment, then exhale slowly.
- Continue this gentle breathing pattern for five cycles.

2. Set Your Gaze

- Close your eyes and set your gaze up at a 45-degree angle as if looking at a point just above your eyebrows.
- This position helps switch your brain into an alpha state, which calms you.
- Keep your eyes focused there as you continue to breathe deeply for a few breaths.

3. Calm Down Your Focus and Brain

- Begin a countdown from 50 to 1, allowing yourself to drift deeper into relaxation with each number.

- By the time you reach 1, you should be in a deeply relaxed state.

4. See Gratitude in the Now
- Visualize something that brings you gratitude now, such as a loved one, a pet, or having a roof over your head.

5. See Gratitude in the Future
- Visualize something you're working toward that you will be grateful for once you beat sleep apnea, such as renewed energy, improved relationships, or the ability to pursue your passions.

6. Transition Back
- Take one more deep breath and slowly open your eyes.
- Feel refreshed, rejuvenated, and ready to embrace the rest of your day with a calm and positive outlook.
- Note how you feel physically, emotionally, and mentally.

By incorporating these practices into your daily routine, you can calm your nervous system, improve your breathing, and enhance your overall sleep quality.

How Do You Know This Is Working?

Just like with most of the action steps in this book, you can start to expect the following:
- Your energy levels remain consistent throughout the day without frequent crashes, suggesting a balanced nervous system.

- You experience fewer and less intense episodes of anxiety or stress, showing that your nervous system is calmer and more regulated.
- You notice a reduction in the frequency and severity of your sleep apnea episodes, indicating improved nervous system function.
- You find it easier to fall asleep and stay asleep through the night, demonstrating a more relaxed and balanced nervous system.
- Your overall mood improves, and you feel more focused and productive, reflecting a well-regulated nervous system.

Roadblocks Ahead

And, of course, life is not always rainbows and unicorns when we set out to accomplish something. So, here are the roadblocks to be aware of:

- **Individual Lifestyle Factors:** Many people have unique lifestyle factors, such as high-stress jobs or irregular schedules, that can keep their nervous system in overdrive. Personalized strategies are essential to address these specific challenges effectively.
- **Personalized Stress Management:** There are many ways to calm the nervous system, such as mindfulness practices or specific exercises.

- **Consistency Issues:** Maintaining consistency in relaxation techniques can be challenging without ongoing support and accountability.
- **Adapting to New Routines:** Forming new habits to calm your nervous system can be difficult.

Wrapping Up This Chapter

In this chapter, we've explored the critical role of the nervous system in sleep apnea and how calming it down can significantly improve your sleep quality and overall health. By understanding and addressing the factors that keep your nervous system in overdrive, you can break the cycle of poor sleep and nerve damage. As you implement these strategies, you'll notice improvements in your energy levels, mood, and sleep patterns. Next, let's talk about the environment!

Exclusive Book Bonus: Gratitude Reset Audio Track

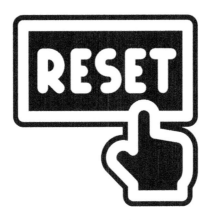

I always find it helpful when I have something easy to follow along with. So, instead of having to memorize the steps of the gratitude reset, I recorded an audio track you can put on your phone to play when needed. Go ahead and use the link below to get it:

TheSleepApneaSolution.com/reset

And, of course, you can also use the QR code below:

Client Highlight: Richard's Journey to Better Sleep

"When I began, I was skeptical about the relaxation protocols you gave me. But, after a few days, this has been a total game changer for my sleep!"

Our client Richard, 66, from Denver, Colorado

For over a decade, Richard struggled with sleep apnea, caught in "CPAP limbo." Despite using his CPAP, he woke up exhausted. Without it, his snoring kept his wife, Eileen, in the guest room. His days were filled with fatigue and naps instead of enjoying retirement. He missed out on playing with his grandkids, which deeply saddened him.

One morning, Richard had to cancel a promised outing with his grandkids because he was too tired. Seeing their disappointment was a wake-up call. He knew he needed to change but was overwhelmed by the thought of trying another solution after many had failed.

Late one night, Richard found hope in our Facebook group, reading about lifestyle-based protocols that helped others. He scheduled a free evaluation call with me, armed with countless questions. During our conversation, I assured him that while this approach required his active participation, it could work if he committed to it.

Richard decided to take the plunge. We discovered that his nervous system was in overdrive from years of disrupted sleep. Initially, Richard struggled with incorporating relaxation techniques into his daily routine, finding it difficult to slow down his racing thoughts. We helped him by introducing simple, manageable practices like guided breathing exercises that he could easily fit into his busy schedule.

By focusing on these relaxation techniques, Richard experienced profound shifts within weeks. His sleep became deeper, and he woke up feeling refreshed. His energy levels improved, and he enjoyed quality time with his grandkids and leisurely strolls with Eileen. This transformation highlighted the importance of calming the nervous system for his nighttime breathing and sleep quality.

As Richard's need for his CPAP faded, he felt liberated and in control of his life again. He stood taller, embracing his role as a revitalized man, husband, and grandfather.

Overcoming Mental Blocks on Your Healing Journey

Healing from sleep apnea isn't just about physical changes—it's also a mental journey. There's not really a great place for this topic in the book. But, since your nervous system is technically part of the mental aspect, I figured I'd put it at the end of this chapter.

The reality is that many times we "know better" but don't "do better." We may be inconsistent, lose motivation, or fall into poor habits like eating bad foods or staying up too late. The fundamental reasons these happen are due to some of the following mental patterns that keep us stuck. Here are a few to recognize and overcome:

1. **Self-Doubt**: You might think, "I've tried everything and nothing works." This kind of thinking can prevent you from fully committing to new strategies. Remember, each step you take brings you closer to better health. It's about persistence and finding what works for you.

2. **Fear of Change**: Change can be scary, even when it's positive. You might worry that new routines will be too difficult or that you'll fail. Focus on small, manageable changes and celebrate your successes along the way. Every little bit helps.

Dylan Petkus

3. **Perfectionism**: You may feel that if you can't do something perfectly, it's not worth doing at all. This mindset can stop you from making progress. Aim for progress, not perfection. Small, consistent efforts can lead to big improvements over time.

4. **Negative Self-Talk**: "I'm never going to get better," or "I'm just not good at this." These thoughts can sabotage your efforts. Practice self-compassion and remind yourself that healing is a journey. Positive affirmations and celebrating small wins can help shift your mindset.

5. **Comparisons**: It's easy to compare your progress to others and feel discouraged. Remember, everyone's journey is unique. Focus on your own path and what you need to do to move forward.

Recognizing these mental blocks and actively working to overcome them is crucial. However, identifying these patterns in yourself and making long-lasting changes can be challenging. In fact, not only do we provide expert guidance for our clients, but we also make sure we provide the coaching they need to get through these roadblocks. That way, people who would have fallen off the bandwagon are able to make consistent progress toward their health goals.

Chapter 9
Environment

One of the most overlooked factors in addressing sleep apnea is the environment. The environment is all the thousands of different factors surrounding you. You can think of it like how a fish is surrounded by water, radioactive waste, and prescriptions drugs that have been flushed down the toilet. Obviously (and hopefully), you're not surrounded by that type of environment. However, every single client I've worked with had major environmental issues that needed to be addressed.

Environmental factors impact sleep apnea by impacting your breathing. Many of these environmental issues will cause inflammation. In turn, this inflammation will narrow your airway, which leads to faster breathing (and, as a result, more airway collapse). While we've already discussed how light at night can negatively impact sleep, there are other environmental triggers to consider:

- Air Quality: Allergens, particulate matter, and cleaning chemicals can irritate your airways and disrupt breathing.
- Heavy Metal Exposure: Heavy metals can negatively affect overall health and sleep quality.
- Noise Pollution: Excessive or persistent noise can interfere with the ability to fall—and stay—asleep.
- Temperature Fluctuations: An uncomfortable bedroom temperature can disrupt the sleep-wake cycle.
- Electromagnetic Fields (EMF): Some individuals may be sensitive to electromagnetic fields, which can affect sleep patterns.

Understanding these triggers and taking steps to mitigate their impact can help promote better breathing and enhance your overall sleep quality.

What the Research Says

Recent studies provide compelling evidence linking environmental factors to the severity of sleep apnea and overall sleep quality:

Air Pollution and Sleep Apnea:
Researchers found that a 10 μg/m³ (very small) increase in PM2.5 (fine particulate matter) was associated with a seventeen percent higher odds of moderate-to-severe sleep apnea.[39] Research has also shown that exposure to

39 Billings ME et al. The Association of Ambient Air Pollution with Sleep Apnea: The Multi-Ethnic Study of Atherosclerosis. Ann Am Thorac Soc. 2019 Mar;16(3):363-370.

higher levels of nitrogen dioxide (NO_2) and sulfur dioxide (SO_2) significantly increased the risk of sleep apnea.[40]

Heavy Metal Exposure and Sleep Disturbances:
Individuals with high levels of arsenic exposure had a 1.52-fold increased risk of sleep disturbances compared to those with the lowest exposure.[41] They've also found that higher blood lead levels were associated with a twenty-five percent increased risk of short sleep duration (<7 hours) in adults.[42]

Noise Pollution and Sleep Quality:
Every increase of ten decibels (dB) in nighttime noise levels was associated with a fourteen percent increased risk of awakening during the night.[43] For instance, aircraft noise exposure was linked to a decrease in REM sleep,

40 Shen YL et al. Association of PM2.5 with sleep-disordered breathing from a population-based study in Northern Taiwan urban areas. Environ Pollut. 2018 Feb;233:109-113.

41 Liu J et al. Air pollution exposure and adverse sleep health across the life course: A systematic review. Environ Pollut. 2020 Jul;262:114263.

42 Chen S et al. The Causal Association Between Blood Lead and Sleep Disorders: Evidence from National Health and Nutrition Examination Survey and Mendelian Randomization Analysis. J Epidemiol Glob Health. 2024 Jun;14(2):462-469.

43 Halperin D. Environmental noise and sleep disturbances: A threat to health? Sleep Sci. 2014 Dec;7(4):209-12.

with a 1.6 percent reduction in REM sleep for every ten dB increase in noise level.[44]

EMF Exposure and Sleep Disturbances:

A review of twenty-three studies concluded that exposure to radiofrequency electromagnetic fields (RF-EMF) from mobile phones was associated with altered sleep patterns, decreased total sleep time, and reduced sleep efficiency.[45]

They've also found that exposure to pulse-modulated RF-EMF before sleep reduced slow-wave activity (SWA) during non-rapid eye movement (NREM) sleep, which is crucial for memory consolidation and brain plasticity.[46]

These studies highlight the significant impact that environmental factors can have on sleep apnea severity and overall sleep quality. One of the most important environments you need to optimize is the environment you sleep in. So, let's talk about some high-level actions you can take today.

---

44 Basner M, Müller U, Elmenhorst EM. Single and combined effects of air, road, and rail traffic noise on sleep and recuperation. Sleep. 2011 Jan 1;34(1):11-23.

45 Halgamuge MN, Skafidas E, Davis D. A meta-analysis of in vitro exposures to weak radiofrequency radiation exposure from mobile phones (1990-2015). Environ Res. 2020 May;184:109227.

46 Schmid MR et al. Sleep EEG alterations: effects of pulsed magnetic fields versus pulse-modulated radio frequency electromagnetic fields. J Sleep Res. 2012 Dec;21(6):620-9.

Prioritize Air Quality

- *Open Windows*: If the outside air is clean and noise isn't an issue, open a window before bedtime to let fresh air in and improve ventilation. This can help reduce indoor pollutants and create a more oxygen-rich environment for better breathing during sleep.

- *Use Air Purifiers*: Consider using an air purifier to filter out allergens, particulate matter, and other pollutants from the air.

- *Avoid Harsh Chemicals:* Use natural cleaning products and avoid synthetic fragrances that can irritate your airways.

Minimize Noise Pollution

- *Rearrange Your Bed*: If noise is a concern, move your bed away from windows or walls shared with noisy areas, and consider using soft earplugs to block out unwanted sounds.

- *Use Earplugs:* Block out unwanted sounds while sleeping with comfortable earplugs.

- *Create Background Noise*: Use a noise machine or fan to create a consistent background sound that masks disruptive noises.

Tech Timeout

- *Ban Electronics:* Remove electronic devices from the bedroom at least sixty minutes before sleep. Screens emit blue light, which can suppress melatonin production, making it harder to fall asleep.
- *Reduce EMF Exposure:* Keep devices out of the sleep space to minimize electromagnetic field (EMF) exposure, contributing to a better sleep environment.

Maintain a Comfortable Temperature

- *Optimize Temperature:* Keep your bedroom at a cooler temperature to support the body's sleep-wake cycle. There's no perfect number for this. Obviously, even if research studies for men in their 20s say sixty-six degrees Fahrenheit is the best, your individual mileage will vary.
- *Bedding Choices:* Choose breathable, moisture-wicking bedding materials to help regulate your body temperature throughout the night.

How Do You Know This Is Working?

General environmental changes can be a bit of a mixed bag. The results of some changes may not be noticeable for months. Other changes may be an overnight success. Either way, here's what you can look forward to:

- You wake up less frequently during the night due to fewer disturbances from light, noise, or temperature changes.
- Your breathing is more regular and less labored, with fewer apnea episodes disrupting your sleep.
- You experience a significant reduction in snoring, allowing you and your partner to sleep more soundly.
- You wake up feeling more refreshed and less groggy, indicating deeper and more restorative sleep.
- You notice fewer respiratory issues, such as congestion or allergies, which can interfere with breathing during sleep.
- Your overall sleep quality improves, with fewer instances of waking up feeling short of breath or gasping for air.

Roadblocks Ahead

Even though you're on the best path, there are always going to be some challenges around the corner. Here are a few to consider:

- **Identifying Key Factors:** There are too many environmental factors to count. We work to find the most important ones to address for each client.

- **Maintaining Consistency:** Keeping your sleep environment optimized can be challenging without ongoing guidance. Consistency in maintaining an ideal sleep environment requires regular adjustments and support.
- **Individual Preferences:** Each person has unique preferences and sensitivities. Tailoring the sleep environment to your specific needs can be complex.
- **Addressing Unseen Issues:** Some environmental issues, such as allergens or subtle noise disturbances, can be hard to identify and manage on your own.

Environmental Mastery

Your sleep environment is one of the most important (most of the time). As you go throughout your day, there are multiple environments you spend time in such as your office, car, a friend's house, etc. And each environment will have many factors to consider that are beyond the scope of this book. Nonetheless, improving your bedroom environment is a great place for you to start.

Wrapping This Chapter Up

Improving your sleep environment can play a significant role in managing sleep apnea and enhancing your overall sleep quality. By prioritizing air quality, minimizing light and noise pollution, taking a tech timeout, and maintaining a comfortable temperature, you can create a more restful and supportive sleep environment. Each small step you take toward optimizing your bedroom can make a big difference in your journey to better sleep and health.

Katherine's Transformation: From Fatigue to Vitality

Changing my sleep conditions had an immediate effect. I started sleeping better almost right away. I had the energy to get things done and enjoy a social life again. It was great to see things getting better so quickly.

Our client Katherine, 61, from Atlanta, Georgia

Katherine had been battling central sleep apnea for over a decade, leaving her perpetually fatigued and her health in rapid decline. Despite countless adjustments to her CPAP machine and trying every alternative treatment, nothing provided consistent relief. Her social life vanished, and even basic tasks became daunting.

A dizzy spell one afternoon was the final push she needed. She discovered our book, sparking a glimmer of hope with its approach based on lifestyle changes. Implementing the action steps, she saw small improvements but soon realized she needed more personalized guidance.

With hope and nerves, Katherine set up a free evaluation call with me. After she enrolled, we identified environmental factors disrupting her sleep and made tailored adjustments. It took a bit of tinkering around with several factors. But, ultimately, after a lot of time together on our Q&A calls, we were able to optimize her home environment.

Soon, Katherine experienced her first solid nights of sleep in ages, gaining energy and reconnecting with friends. Her self-confidence grew as she began living life fully again.

Over several months, Katherine's sleep efficiency and quality continued to improve. For the first time in over a decade, she fell asleep quickly and woke up rejuvenated. She even lowered her CPAP setting without increased apnea events.

No longer defined by sleep apnea, Katherine felt vibrant and unstoppable. Her days were filled with energy for hikes and new passions. Optimizing key factors transformed her sleep and life incredibly, proving the power of personalized, holistic approaches to health.

Fundamental Bedroom Environment Upgrades

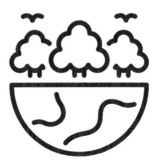

Environmental engineers have checklists to make sure they don't miss anything…

… so, shouldn't you have a checklist too?

That's why I made an easy PDF checklist to download so you can hit the high points from the chapter (and a few more).

Use the link below to get it:

TheSleepApneaSolution.com/environment

As usual, please scan the QR code, if you prefer:

Help Us Help You!

As you've gone through this book and gained tons of insights and action steps, I would love to know how you've been doing! All you need to do is fill out this short survey and I'll give you a free gift! Just use the link below:

TheSleepApneaSolution.com/thanks

Or, please scan the QR code below:

Chapter 10
This is Just the Beginning

Congratulations! You've made it to the end of this book, and I hope you've found the information and strategies to be both enlightening and empowering. By now, you have a good foundation for how sleep apnea can be tackled naturally through a holistic approach to health.

But this is just the beginning of your journey to better sleep and overall well-being. Now that you have the foundation, it's time to take your progress to the next level.

Accelerating your healing journey is essential because that's what will allow you to wake up feeling truly refreshed and ready to tackle the day with enthusiasm. You'll be excited when you can get rid of your CPAP, mouthguard, or any of those band-aids. Time and time again, when our clients do that, it is like declaring victory against sleep apnea.

But that's just the beginning because, remember, this isn't just about sleeping better; this is about living better. You deserve to have the alertness and energy to complete tasks with ease and efficiency. You can reclaim a full life with your family, enjoying spontaneous weekend getaways or lively game nights. And, of course, when you overcome sleep apnea, that's when you can look forward to the next twenty-plus years without worrying about your health.

To help you achieve these outcomes and more, I'm inviting you to an exclusive masterclass. This is your opportunity to learn how to build on the foundation you've established and accelerate your progress dramatically. Here's what you'll get from this masterclass:

Gain In-Depth Knowledge: Receive detailed insights into the underlying causes of sleep apnea and how to address them effectively.

Accelerate Your Progress: Discover advanced strategies that will empower you to speed up your journey to better sleep.

Achieve Lasting Results: Learn how to solidify the changes you've made and ensure long-term success.

This masterclass is not just an extension of the book; it's an opportunity to engage with advanced content and gain valuable insights.

Click the link below or type it into your web browser to access:

TheSleepApneaSolution.com/masterclass

Or, feel free to scan the QR code below if you prefer:

Work With Us

When we first released this book, we got multiple emails and calls per day all asking one question: *"How can I work with you?"* To make it easier for both of us, I'll outline the process here.

The first step is our complimentary 45-minute evaluation session. We offer this because it is beyond frustrating to see a doctor or specialist for your sleep, get asked eight questions, and then just get a recommendation for a CPAP.

Instead, we want to help you gain insights around different aspects of your health so you can make better decisions on your healing journey. That's why in this session, we will:

- Clarify your unique issues and needs
- Determine your goals
- Figure out how to help you achieve them
- If we feel we can help, then we can also discuss what our services look like.

By the end of this call, you will walk away with a new level of hope and a clear direction for your healing journey. This session is focused entirely on you and your needs, giving you personalized insights that you can't get from a book alone.

Now, as awesome as that sounds, this session is ***not*** for everyone.

- If you are someone who thinks overcoming sleep apnea is not worth the effort, then this is *not* for you.
- If you are someone who only wants something covered by insurance, then this is *not* for you.
- If you are someone who is mostly okay with needing a machine to breathe at night, then this is *not* for you.
- If you are someone who accepts pushing through life, then this is *not* for you.

But this session could be a perfect fit if this sounds like you:

- You're someone who *refuses* to go one more night with a device or snoring that makes sleep a hassle for you (and your partner).
- You're someone who *must* resurrect their productivity for projects at work and home.
- You're someone who *must* reclaim your role as an engaged, energetic parent or grandparent who makes every moment count.
- You're someone who *must* regain your passion and joy for sharing adventures with your partner.
- You're someone who *must* recapture an active lifestyle that fulfills you.
- You're *willing to* take guidance from an expert and *take action*.

If the above sounds like you, then this session is for you.

If you are ready, please click here or go to TheSleepApneaSolution.com/chat to schedule your free evaluation call. Fill out the initial application, and then book your time to connect with myself or a member of our staff.

Of course, here's the QR code if it's easier to scan with your phone or tablet:

Thank you for reading, and I look forward to speaking with you soon,

Dylan Petkus, MD, MPH, MS

Case Studies To Inspire You

Navigating your journey with sleep apnea can sometimes feel like an uphill climb, but seeing the success of others can provide that extra spark of motivation we all need. That's why we've gathered a few incredible success stories that we'd love to share with you. These are real stories from real people who have made significant strides in their battle against poor sleep. We hope these stories inspire you to stay consistent and keep pushing forward.

Ready to be inspired? Just click the link below or scan the QR code to dive into these amazing journeys:

TheSleepApneaSolution.com/results

Thank You For Reading!

Thank you for reading! If this book has helped you in any way, please take a moment to give us feedback via the link below. Any insights you provide will help us help more people who struggle with sleep apnea. And, for your feedback, we'll give you a free gift! So, kindly click or type the link below into your browser:

TheSleepApneaSolution.com/thanks

And, if you prefer to use a QR code, here it is:

Printed in Great Britain
by Amazon

55607247R00116